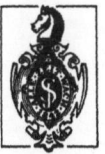

Roger Eltringham · Michael Durkin
Sue Andrewes · William Casey

Post-anaesthetic Recovery

A Practical Approach

Second Edition

Foreword by Luke M. Kitahata

With 38 Figures

Springer-Verlag
London Berlin Heidelberg New York
Paris Tokyo Hong Kong

Roger Eltringham, MB, ChB, FFARCS
Michael Durkin, MB, BS, FFARCS
William Casey, MB, ChB, FFARCS
Consultant Anaesthetists, Gloucestershire Royal Hospital,
Great Western Road, Gloucester GL1 3NN, UK

Sue Andrewes RGN, RSCN
Formerly Nursing Officer, Recovery Unit,
Whipps Cross Hospital, London E11 1NR, UK

ISBN–13:978–3–540–19555–9

British Library Cataloguing in Publication Data
Eltringham, Roger
Post-anaesthetic recovery.—2nd ed.
1. Medicine. Anaesthesia. Monitoring   I. Eltringham, Roger 617'.96
ISBN–13:978–3–540–19555–9   e–ISBN–13:978–1–4471–1693–6
DOI: 10.1007/978–1–4471–1693–6

Library of Congress Cataloging-in-Publication Data
Post-anaesthetic recovery: a practical approach/Roger Eltringham . . . [et al.];
foreword by Luke M. Kitahata.—2nd ed.
p. cm. Rev. ed. of: Post-anaesthetic recovery/Roger Eltringham, Michael Durkin,
Sue Andrewes. 1983.   Includes bibliographies and index.
ISBN–13:978–3–540–19555–9 (U.S.)
1. Anesthesia—Complications and sequelae. 2. Postoperative care. I. Eltringham,
Roger, 1939–   . [DNLM: 1. Anesthesia—nurses' instruction. 2. Postoperative
Care—nurses' instruction. 3. Postoperative Complications—prevention & control—
nurses' instruction. 4. Recovery Room—nurses' instruction. WY 154 P857]
RD82.5.P67 1989 617'.919—dc19 DNLM/DLC.
for Library of Congress   89–6032
                                                                          CIP

© Springer-Verlag Berlin Heidelberg 1983, 1989
First published 1983; Second edition 1989

The use of registered names, trademarks etc. in this publication does not imply, even
in the absence of a specific statement, that such names are exempt from the relevant
laws and regulations and therefore free for general use.

Product Liability: The publisher can give no guarantee for information about drug
dosage and application thereof contained in this book. In every individual case the
respective user must check its accuracy by consulting other pharmaceutical literature.

Filmset by Macmillan India Limited, Bangalore 560 025

2128/3916–54321   Printed on acid-free paper

To Lorna Eltringham,
Richard Andrewes
and
Sue Durkin

Foreword to the Second Edition

The need for continued vigilance in the post-anaesthetic recovery period following general or regional anaesthesia is paramount. This book brings together in one volume the major issues that one should consider in the management of the patient during this period.

Improvements in modern surgical techniques continue to stimulate great advances in anaesthetic management. Large groups of patients who until recently would not have been candidates for surgery are now able to benefit from such surgery because of improved knowledge of anaesthetic pharmacology, the physiology of pain transmission and cardiopulmonary monitoring.

The first chapter concentrates on the organisation of the recovery room; it deals with management from the standpoint of the United Kingdom but is equally applicable to the rest of the world. The nursing and medical procedures for normal recovery are discussed in Chapter 2. In the later chapters there is a comprehensive review of complications in the post-anaesthetic period and a discussion of specific aspects of recovery from specialised surgical procedures. Finally, a unique chapter deals with the pre-operative factors that will affect the recovery period. Additions to the first edition include chapters covering methods of pain relief, day case surgery and the various monitoring techniques now available for use in the recovery room.

The authors have succeeded in bringing together a rational plan for the management of many problems which routinely affect a patient's recovery from anaesthesia. They have done this in a problem-solving fashion with the emphasis on reaching a management decision as a result of careful clinical examination and monitoring. It is evident that all personnel involved in the recovery of the patient from anaesthesia need a concise, clinical and relevant book from which they can obtain advice. There is no doubt that this is just such a book, and it will provide for nurses, doctors and all those involved in the field a practical guide to this often neglected critical period following anaesthesia.

Luke M. Kitahata, MD, PhD
Professor of Anesthesiology
Yale University, USA

Preface to the Second Edition

Developments in surgery have enabled more ambitious operations to be attempted than ever before, while similar advances in anaesthesia and monitoring have meant that many patients who were previously considered unfit now undergo surgery.

It is essential that standards of patient care during surgery are continued post-operatively until the depressant effects of anaesthesia have worn off and it is safe for patients to return to the wards or to their homes. The importance of adequate supervision by well-trained nursing staff in properly equipped surroundings has been recognised by the introduction of recovery rooms in most hospitals. Despite this, many patients still emerge from anaesthesia in wards or departments where they are supervised by inexperienced nursing staff in unfamiliar surroundings.

Recovery from anaesthesia may be accompanied by a variety of dangerous and potentially fatal complications, many of which can be avoided by the detection of early warning signs and the institution of appropriate therapy before an irreversible situation is allowed to develop.

This book describes the major complications liable to be encountered and suggests how they may be avoided by careful monitoring, vigilant nursing and sound organisation. The patient's behaviour at recovery is influenced by his pre-operative condition, by drug therapy pre- and intra-operatively and by the nature of the surgery, and sections have been devoted to these aspects since a basic understanding of them is essential in anticipating events in the recovery room.

In this second edition, there is a chapter on pain management that includes information on both the advantages and the problems that may be encountered when local anaesthetic blocks are used. There are also new chapters on the special considerations that apply to recovery nursing in day care units and on the role of monitoring equipment in the recovery room.

Throughout the text drugs have been referred to by their British Pharmacopoeia name with the US equivalent in parentheses when this is different. In Appendix A common brand names are also included.

For clarity, throughout this book, it is assumed that patients and doctors are male and that nurses are female. No slight is intended to members of either gender, and we trust no one will be offended by this usage.

It is hoped that this book will provide a readily available source of practical information not only for nursing staff but also for junior anaesthetists and house surgeons and for all those involved in the care of patients in the immediate post-operative period.

Acknowledgements

The authors are indebted to their many medical and nursing colleagues in Bristol, Gloucester and at Whipps Cross Hospital, London for their help and encouragement in the preparation of this work. In particular we appreciate the help given by Tony Bennett, Geoffrey Burton, Paul Thornton and Sheila Willatts, consultant anaesthetists from Bristol, and Mike Gear and Reggie Merryweather, consultant surgeons, Philip Kingston, consultant haematologist, and Steve Wilkinson, consultant physician, all from Gloucester and to Lynda Taylor for infection control update.

We are grateful to Patricia Stone, Marion Heath and Jean Blake, all pharmacists, for their painstaking work in checking the drug names and their American equivalents, to Steve Catchpole and Sue Durkin for the illustrations, and to Dick Andrewes for repeatedly typing the manuscripts and indexing.

We express also our gratitude to Michael Jackson and Wendy Darke of Springer-Verlag and to the late and very sadly missed John Farman of Addenbrooke's Hospital, Cambridge, for their helpful advice throughout the preparation of the manuscript.

Finally, a special word of thanks is due to Prof. Harold Carron of the University of Virginia who offered invaluable advice during the preparation of this work and whom we failed to acknowledge in the first edition. Our sincere apologies and grateful thanks.

Gloucester and Loughton   Roger Eltringham
1989   Michael Durkin
                                                Sue Andrewes
                                                William Casey

Contents

Chapter 1
Organisation

Role of the Recovery Room

The Recovery Room is an area within the operating theatre unit where short-term critical care is given after surgery and anaesthesia. It is here that support is provided for the patient through the reversing stages of anaesthesia until he is fully conscious, his protective reflexes have returned and his vital signs are stable.

It is at this time that the patient is vulnerable to many complications especially those which are respiratory or circulatory in origin. Farman (1978) reports that 1 in 5.5 patients showed problems after anaesthesia and surgery. Eltringham (1979) reports similar figures. The College of Anaesthetists and the Association of Anaesthetists of Great Britain and Ireland have made recommendations on staffing in recovery areas and facilities that should be available to all patients. It is disconcerting to learn that a recent survey has shown that one third of patients who died within six days of surgery did not have the benefit of adequate recovery facilities. These statistics alone justify having a special holding area. Additionally, the statement is made (Atkinson et al. 1982) that "about 20% of deaths associated with anaesthesia occur in the first 30 minutes after operation". This shows clearly how potentially hazardous this time can be. The real value of a recovery service in closely monitoring the patient and treating problems as they arise, thus preventing them from becoming life-threatening should now be clear to all.

This service should be provided with a satisfactory site and the equipment necessary for routine and emergency use. It should be staffed by nurses experienced in the use of this equipment and trained in all aspects of monitoring the patient throughout his stay. Then, with the sanction of the anaesthetist, the patient would be returned to his ward fully conscious and with his vital signs stable.

Site

The correct site for the recovery room is adjoining the operating theatre or theatres it serves, although this important feature has not always been recognised in planning large units. The architect may have considered the seemingly rational scheme of following the patient's progress in the operating theatre suite with the recovery room at the end of the "production line" and next to the exit. The main consideration is always to have it in close proximity to the operating theatre it serves.

To site it without easy access to the operating theatre is to ignore the nature of the nursing carried out in the recovery room and the need for the anaesthetist to review easily his patient's post-anaesthetic progress, He may require to start corrective or emergency treatment without delay. Nursing staff may often require immediate help or advice, the time factor being of paramount significance.

The second important reason for having the shortest possible route between operating theatre and recovery room is the potential risk involved in the transport of an unconscious patient. After his full recovery and when sanction has been given for his return to the ward, he may be transferred a longer distance with safety.

Reception Area

Reception wards are planned in many operating theatre entrances. Here the patient rests until the anaesthetist is ready to receive him. In the planning of some theatre units a holding bay is incorporated allowing for timed pre-anaesthetic medications to be given. The lights may be dimmed and quiet should be maintained. Manning of this area by the recovery nurses introduces a valuable time for the collection of individual data on each patient. This charted information, essential both for the recovery nurse and the anaesthetist, will then form the base line of knowledge to be used at the patient's recovery time and will provide continuity of the patient's ward care plan.

Though the entrance and exit of an operating theatre unit can share the same porterage and hand-over resources, it should be designed so that an incoming patient does not meet a returning post-operative patient.

The terms "clean" or "dirty", "sterile" or "unsterile area", refer to their position in relation to the demarcation barrier for the operating theatre unit. Across this barrier regulations must exist for clothing, footwear and antistatic precautions. The post-anaesthetic recovery room is thus sited within the boundaries of these theatre regulations so that there is complete freedom of movement for all staff working in recovery. A unit outside, i.e. in the unsterile/dirty area is described by Renfrew and McManus (1975). This is not the custom generally in Great Britain. A 24-hour recovery service described as an Acute Care Unit with 22 beds is in operation at the Nuffield Orthopaedic Centre, Oxford (Wakeley 1974). This is situated outside the operating theatres in the unsterile area though an integral part of the operating theatre complex.

Relationship with an Intensive Therapy Unit

It is an advantage to have an intensive therapy unit (ITU) and operating theatre unit on the same floor level and adjacent to one another. A direct door access is not advised, as operating theatre infection control measures are difficult to enforce at such an entrance. An agreed policy of acceptance of a patient by ITU should exist.

Windows

An architectural feature of value is the provision of windows on an outside wall. An outlook on the world and the natural lighting this affords can compensate for the possible tensions of the work.

Design

Number of Bays

The number of equipped bays in the recovery room will be dictated by the type of surgery undertaken. The Department of Health and Social Security advises that three bays are sufficient for general surgery in a twin operating theatre unit (DHSS 1975). In practice it has been found that more bays are required because provision must also be made for the occasional need to accommodate a patient requiring intermittent positive pressure ventilation (IPPV) after operation. This special bay must have more space and needs to be similar in size to the measurements laid down by ITU standards (DHSS 1974).

Theatres in which large numbers of short operations are performed, e.g. gynaecological and ear, nose and throat surgery, should have available at least three bays per operating theatre (Hudson 1979). It must be remembered that short operations do not necessarily mean trouble-free and equally short recovery periods. A large recovery room serving five to ten theatres can allow for a more economic use of space. For a unit of eight theatres, 12 bed spaces in recovery were found to be sufficient (Farman 1978).

If ketamine hydrochloride or other cataleptic anaesthetics are to be used for children and adults, a bay should be provided where quiet may be maintained. A "Ketalar" blue disc is affixed to bed or trolley to indicate that the patient must not be disturbed (Clark 1973, Hollister and Burn 1974).

It must be thought of as the patient's right to be allocated a space for his recovery time. The number of equipped and staffed bays should always be sufficient even if under-utilised at times.

Space per Bed

The floor space needed per bed or per trolley will be 9.5 m^2 (approximately 100 ft^2). For the bay used for IPPV support, 18.5 m^2 (approximately 200 ft^2)

will be required. When the bays are placed opposite each other, enough clearance must be allowed in the centre of the unit for the easy movement of patients, 1.7 m (5.5 ft) is sufficient.

Whether to use beds or trolleys will depend upon the working plans of the operating theatre suite. In newer hospitals, mobile ward beds are commonly transferred to the recovery room. They are suitable only if they can produce the following features:

1. A two-way tilt, Trendelenburg and reverse
2. Folding side rails
3. Back-rest support
4. Fore-and-aft wheel-locking devices
5. Fore-and-aft sites for infusion poles

The bed head must be removable to allow for full control of the patient's head and airway.

Trolleys must have the above characteristics plus a transfer-top to align with the outside trolley. They should have deep firm mattresses. The base of these trolleys should be X-ray translucent and incorporate a cassette-holder of chest X-ray size.

Lighting

Lighting standards may be critical in recovery areas. Accurate assessment of the patient's central and peripheral colour is a significant monitoring variant. Distortion can be caused by the colour characteristics of the light source and also by reflection from the walls. Decoration of recovery areas should be in soft colours other than greens or blues. Fluorescent lighting is economical and the tubes should have a colour temperature of 4000K. Exacting procedures such as the institution of a central venous pressure (CVP) line may require an additional and mobile light source. Lighting in recovery areas should always be included on the emergency lighting circuit.

It should be remembered that the patient emerging from anaesthesia may be subjected to considerable glare from overhead lights. It is useful to have light-dimming facilities for the benefit of patients emerging from cataleptic-type, e.g. ketamine anaesthesia.

Power Outlet Points

The number of sockets at each patient's bay should be sufficient to power all the electrical equipment that may be required. There should be at least four outlets per bay. Any of the following apparatus may be required:

1. Blood warmer
2. Electrocardiogram (ECG)
3. Mobile light
4. Incubator

5. D.C. defibrillator
6. Pressure monitor screen
7. Syringe pump

Additional outlets should be provided for the IPPV bay since a ventilator will require a further power socket. Provision should be made for the use of X-ray machines and an X-ray viewing screen.

Communication Systems

The best system in the past, and it still has much worth, is a great yell from the nurse. However, since greater distances reduce the success of this method of alerting people to recovery problems, emergency bells or intercom systems have been supplied. It is always important to test any electronic alarm circuit at the commencement of the day as part of the cockpit drill of all emergency equipment. The intercom two-way call system should be at each patient's bay. To leave any patient's side at a critical time in order to attract help is to jeopardise further the patient's safety. Staff should not be left to work on their own in the recovery unit, either at the end of surgical lists or at night.

A single operating theatre will not need this two-way communication system if the recovery area is adjacent to the theatre but an emergency bell to call for assistance is still a vital piece of equipment.

Any call system should not be relayed to an anaesthetic room direct. It could disturb induction of anaesthesia, when quiet is an important factor. The call can be transmitted to the theatre or a visual signal may be used. Alarms should additionally communicate with all staff rest rooms.

Telephones

There are good grounds for having a telephone which only conducts outgoing calls, in-coming calls being handled by a receptionist outside the recovery area. The persistent ringing of phones and the consequent need to answer them constitute an unnecessary distraction. Again, to leave the side of a recovery patient in order to deal with a call is a potentially dangerous practice.

Noise Levels

Recovery Rooms should be designated "quiet areas". Remembering that a patient's hearing is the first of his senses to return at the anaesthetic reversing time, a noisy environment is undesirable. Shouting at a patient should never be necessary in conveying a command. The careful listening needed for the monitoring of the patient's breathing performance and for blood pressure monitoring is difficult against a background of noise. To design an entrance or exit of a recovery room so that staff can congregate and parley there is unsuitable. As at a party, the volume of noise can rise to unacceptable levels unbeknownst to the perpetrators.

All equipment on wheels should be regularly serviced so that they perform correctly and silently.

Heating and Ventilation

The patient must be received into an area as warm as the operating theatre from which he has come. Since significant heat loss may have occurred in the operating theatre, especially during prolonged surgery and at the extremes of age, further heat dissipation by a low ambient temperature in the recovery room is prejudicial to the patient's progress. A room temperature of 23–24 °C (73–75 °F) with a relative humidity of 50%–60% is satisfactory. There should be a minimum of six changes of air per hour (DHSS 1975) but to increase this rate will bring in an undesirable air-flow chill factor. Additional radiators are always useful for the warming of patient's linen. See also hypothermia/heat loss page 98.

Equipment

The equipment of the recovery area can be divided for convenience into four groups:

1. The basic equipment needed for every patient
2. Respiratory support equipment
3. Cardiovascular support equipment
4. Special nursing and diagnostic equipment

1. *Basic equipment, preferably wall mounted*
    a) Twin oxygen outlets with flowmeters. The first for the administration of humidified oxygen via clear vinyl face mask, nasal cannulae or T-piece system. The second to incorporate a Mapleson C circuit with anaesthetic mask (Fig. 2.14). Mobile oxygen cylinders are required in the event of pipeline failure.
    b) A suction unit with vacuum regulator and sterilisable collection jars plus a full range of suction catheters and Yankauer suction unions. A mobile foot-operated suction machine is required in case of vacuum line failure
    c) Sphygmomanometer with cuff selection, e.g. infant, paediatric, adult and obese and a stethoscope with diaphragm end. (Staff should be advised to provide their own stethoscopes).
    d) Shelf for water bowl, swabs, small dressings, receiver (vomit bowl), disposable container for used needles, clipboard for individual recovery charts, boom or drip stands. There should be a shelf for extra pillows, blankets and aluminium foil space blankets, mobile light and waste disposal bins.

2. *Respiratory support equipment*
Range of oropharyngeal and nasopharyngeal airways
Face masks
Ambu bag
Laryngoscopes with spare blades, batteries and bulbs
Complete range of endotracheal tubes and introducers
Magill forceps
Syringe for cuff inflation with tube-clamping forceps
Bandage and strapping to secure endotracheal tubes
Catheter mounts
Mechanical ventilator
Anaesthetic machine
Wright respirometer
Paediatric anaesthetic set including tubes, masks and laryngoscope
Chest drain equipment
Crico-thyroid puncture set
Ferguson mouth gag
Bronchoscope
Incubator for neonates
Cylinder containing helium 80% and oxygen 20%. A correct pin index post
will be required
Pulse oximeter and capnograph

3. *Cardiovascular support equipment*
Intravenous infusion sets and cannulae (adult and infant)
Blood warmer
Pressure infusor
Blood filters
Central venous cannulae and manometer
Intravenous cut down set
ECG electrodes
Monitor for ECG and blood pressure display and write-out facility
Defibrillator with synchronisation adaptor
Oesophageal or trans-venous pacing equipment
Pressure transducers, transcutaneous oxygen monitor
Doppler ultrasonic device

4. *Nursing and diagnostic equipment*
Bladder irrigation equipment
Urine drainage bags with measuring jug
Surgical dressing pack and pads (gynaecology)
Thermometers (oral, rectal and low reading)

Hyperthermia pack

Range of syringes and needles

Specimen bottles for Hb, electrolytes, cross matching, clotting studies and blood sugar

Dextrostix and Reflomat

Litmus paper

Peripheral nerve stimulator

Warming lamp

Fan

Clock with second sweep hand

Volumetric infusion pumps

5. *Drugs.* The recovery unit will require a wide range of drugs. The most commonly used are listed in Appendix A. There should be a Controlled Drugs cupboard in the recovery room.

Safety

Pollution

It has been well documented that contamination by anaesthetic agents is not confined, as was first thought, to the operating theatre. It has been found that unacceptable pollutant levels of nitrous oxide and halothane are exhaled by the patient post-operatively. A measure of up to 1000 parts per million (ppm) of nitrous oxide near the head of the patient in recovery can be regarded as typical (Howorth 1980). Safety levels have been set for nitrous oxide at 25–30 ppm and for halothane at 0.5 ppm. The recovery personnel are therefore at as much risk as their colleagues in the operating theatre.

Scavenging systems, either active or passive, are now in use in operating theatres for the ducting of anaesthetic agents away from the patient. They are dependent for their correct functioning on the collection of expired gases from the anaesthetic circuit. This same system cannot be applied to the recovery area where the anaesthetic circuit is no longer in use and the patient is exhaling into the atmosphere. The prime concerns of those caring for him at this time is maintenance of his airway and unrestricted access to the patient. Of necessity, the staff will be in close proximity to his exhalations and it is here that the gas pollution levels are at their highest.

A solution to this problem has been described by Howorth (1980). The scavenging system applicable to recovery areas requires an active exhauster power unit (EXFLOW). To this is connected a wide bore tube mounted on a boom for each patient site. The tube terminates in a collecting funnel which is positioned over the patient's nose and mouth. The practicality of its use needs to be reviewed by senior recovery personnel. Its installation cost would be a deciding factor for each Health Authority. The plan for its use would be brought into new theatre design at the operational policy phase, which is the architect's briefing stage.

A face mask incorporating activated charcoal as an adsorbtion barrier to the inhalation of anaesthetic vapours is under investigation. Nitrous oxide concentration cannot, however, be reduced by this method.

The DHSS health circular (76) 38 advises that steps should be taken to reduce levels of pollution in operating departments. The Health Authorities are reminded of their obligation under the Health and Safety at Work Act to provide a safe working environment. Although informing and counselling of staff about these risks are always advised [DHSS HC (76) 38, Appendix 1], a more positive approach must be adopted. It is no longer acceptable to protect staff in one part of an operating theatre unit and ignore another known vulnerable area such as the recovery room.

Fire Risk

A fire depends on three factors:

1. A flammable substance
2. A supply of oxygen
3. A source of ignition

A fire could start in the recovery room as all three factors could be present at the same time as a result of carelessness:

1. The spillage of a spirit-based liquid or a volatile anaesthetic fluid
2. Oxygen therapy in use
3. A spark generated by the build-up of static electricity from unsuitable patient covering, staff clothing or faulty electrical equipment. Total restrictions on smoking in the recovery room must, of course, be strictly observed.

The elements which lead to combustion or explosion must be understood. From senior staff to the most junior ancillary worker, all should be required to attend fire-fighting lectures annually.

Infection Control and Staff Protection

In a post-anaesthetic recovery unit, multiple patient care is undertaken, so that the potential risk of infection and cross-infection could, as a consequence, be high. Any departure from good nursing standards will be seen in an increased rate of post-operative infection on the surgical wards. The patient's time in the recovery room is too short to be able to note this problem. Guidelines for the management of infection control must involve the hospital's Infection Control Nurse, the Central Sterile Supply Department, the Theatre Sterile Supply Unit, the Microbiology Department and the Pharmacy Department. Risk factors will be identified and the precautions to be undertaken will be listed. Protocols for nursing infectious patients will be laid down.

Any advice should certainly start with the simple, if basic, requirement that all medical and nursing staff should wash their hands before and after attending a patient. No longer can it be allowed that medical status thereby confers immunity to pathological laws. We all have an obligation not only to our patients but to ourselves in this matter.

Policies constantly require review. Formerly we were able to prevent known infective patients, e.g. gas gangrene and diagnosed Hepatitis B Virus (HBV) patients, from being admitted to recovery units, their recovery taking place in the operating theatre. The inexorable spread of AIDS means that increasing numbers of undiagnosed patients with Human Immunodeficiency Virus (HIV) and unidentified HBV may potentially be included in all surgical lists, with attendant risks to both medical and nursing staff.

Advice to staff must now include the wearing of protective clothing. The involvement of patients' body fluids, in particular the irrigation of bladders and the vaginal inspection of gynaecological operation sites, will need planned procedures. In cases of dental, oral, nose and throat operations, when the coughing of blood-stained fluid is a possibility, staff must protect themselves with masks, goggles and visors. In dental practice, recommendations to personnel are well defined and pertinent to post-anaesthetic recovery (PAR) units. (Dinsdale 1985).

The re-use of any disposable equipment for economic reasons must now be discontinued. Syringe and needle sets where the point of the needle is guarded to prevent needle-stick may be introduced. The action of resheathing needles is a potentially dangerous one and the DHSS specification for the disposal of used needles and syringes must be adhered to (DHSS TTS/5/330015).

Precautions for the handling of linen, specimens and PAR equipment must be covered by a defined policy.

If patients arrive with a known history of open pulmonary tuberculosis it is a wise precaution that equipment used during anaesthesia accompanies them to the recovery unit. The attending staff should use disposable gloves. Used disposable equipment should be sealed in a colour-coded bag and sent for incineration. The anaesthetic equipment should be autoclaved.

If a patient has an infected wound site or is incontinent of faeces or urine, the trolley or bed should be protected with non-porous disposable drapes. After use, the trolley should be withdrawn and washed and the rubber mattress disinfected with a strong hypochlorite solution and thoroughly dried before being re-issued.

Advice for Recovery Staff

The following is an example of an advice form which could be issued to new staff working in recovery:

1. *Pollution by anaesthetic gases* exhaled by patients in their recovery time. At special risk are female staff contemplating becoming pregnant or in their first trimester when the risk of miscarriage is greater. Please notify the head of department if these circumstances apply.

2. *Fire and explosion risks*
   a) Combustion risk. Oxygen at high flow rates is frequently used during the recovery period.
   b) Explosive risks. Volatile anaesthetic fluids should never be used as cleaning agents for equipment.
   c) Pressurised medical gas cylinders should be handled with care. They should be properly racked, mounted on wall brackets or mobile stands.
   d) Anti-static clothing and footwear should conform to operating theatre standards.
   e) Fire regulations should be read and the instructions acted upon. Attend the fire-fighting lectures yearly.
   f) The positions of assembly points, fire-doors and exits should be known.
   g) The positions and use of fire-extinguishers and their colour coding should be known.
   h) The positions of fire alarms and fire-hosing sites should be known.
3. *X-rays.* Evacuation of the immediate vicinity is recommended during exposure time. If the nurse has to remain with the patient, a protective lead apron should be worn.
4. *Protection of staff.* Staff are advised to wear gloves for their own protection, changing them between patients and especially when:
   a) Handling strong chemical fluids
   b) Handling open blood unit packs
   c) Undertaking bladder irrigation procedures
   d) Inspecting soiled pads and dressing areas or changing soiled linen and handling patient's specimens
   e) Contaminated spillages are being cleared
   Staff should wear gloves whenever they have open cuts or abrasions and occlusive waterproof dressings should be used.
5. *Health.* Staff who are suffering from any infection should report the fact to senior staff.
6. *Lifting and handling of patients.* Correct turning techniques should be learnt so that back strain is minimised.
7. *Restless and violent patients.* Nursing staff should seek help by using the emergency call bell rather than attempt to control these patients single-handed.
8. *Accidents* should be reported to the senior staff and recorded in the appropriate manner. This should include injuries caused by sharp equipment, needles, etc. Witnesses should also make a signed statement.
9. *Defective equipment.* For the protection of all staff and patients, any defective piece of equipment must at once be withdrawn from use and labelled. No adaptations or attempts to mend equipment are allowed. It should at once be brought to the attention of senior staff.
10. *HBV vaccination* is now widely available and staff are urged to be protected in this way. Three doses are needed with a check of antibody levels within one year.
    Sound advice to all recovery staff. Never work in ignorance. If you do not know, ask. If you are not sure, confirm. Remember that good communication is the essence of safety.

Anti-static Precautions

Anti-static precautions are only required where flammable anaesthetics are to be administered. This is seldom the case in recovery areas. If they are required, breathing circuits must be of anti-static rubber and conductive footwear should be worn. Floors should be dampened (p. 13).

Any equipment common to both recovery unit and operating theatre will need to conform to all anti-static requirements. If medical and nursing staff have access to both areas then their footwear and clothing must be in accordance with anti-static regulations.

Switches and sockets, regardless of their fixing height, do not have to be of a sparkless type (DHSS 1969).

Routine cleaning

Clear instruction should be written for daily or weekly cleaning and sterilising of every piece of recovery equipment. Every sterilising routine should commence with a cleaning process. This consists of a wash with clean water, followed by a hot detergent, which in itself eliminates a high proportion of microbes and some bacterial spores. If a disinfectant solution is being used its strength should be exact and not left to guesswork. Finally, a thorough rinsing should take place and the article left to dry. The growth of pathogens, e.g. *Pseudomonas sp.* is always more likely on wet surfaces than on dry. Suction jars should therefore be left dry, as a disinfectant solution, however reassuring it may look, can soon become contaminated in a warm atmosphere.

Equipment which is part of an inspiratory circuit must be carefully examined to eliminate the possibility of a patient breathing in particles of fibre, fluff or fluids left behind in the cleaning process. These could be inhaled into the lungs at an early stage of recovery when the patient's cough reflex is still absent.

All equipment in a recovery unit must either be able to be sterilised or be disposable. Introduction of new equipment should include learning the manufacturer's instructions on how to maintain, clean and sterilise it. Such mundane articles as blood pressure cuffs should not escape the scrutiny of the nurse. They could well be a source of infection. Manufacturers could, with advantage, produce them in a light colour rather than black.

Cleaning materials themselves may be a source of microbial spread. They should either be disposable or recycled daily through a laundering or autoclaving process. Only concentrated solutions of disinfectants should be stored.

Flooring

The flooring of recovery areas should have the following characteristics:

1. Hard-wearing properties and ability to support heavy wheeled equipment without damage to its surface
2. Quiet to the tread of anti-static clogs and sandals
3. A surface inpervious to water and spilled liquids

4. Readily cleanable

5. No shrinkage at joining areas

Vinyl floors satisfy these requirements.

Cleaning. Small spills should be removed at once before they dry. Larger contaminated spillages may be covered with a sodium hypochlorite solution 1%, or with absorbent granules and powders designed for this purpose.

The floor should be wet mopped at least once a day with the minimum quantity of a cold water and detergent solution. Vinyl floors may be polished with a water-emulsion polish. Solvent-based cleaners and polishes should not be used.

It is important that mop heads, whether of cotton or plastic, should be washed daily and then sent for autoclaving or pasteurising (temperature 65 °C, i.e. 149 °F held for 10 minutes). Alternatively, the hospital laundry service may be used for a daily rotation of cleaned mop heads. The use of chemical disinfection agents is not a satisfactory method.

Anti-static flooring is seldom a recommendation for the recovery unit. It is therefore well to have a warning notice to this effect so that it will be clear to the anaesthetist that further precautions must be taken if flammable agents are to be used. In particular the floor should be dampened within touching distance of the patient's breathing circuit with water and detergent.

Equipment Disinfection and Sterilisation

Equipment made of rubber or plastic and not incorporating metal may be sterilised in a freshly made-up solution of hypochlorite 1 : 80 (1.25%), i.e. 100 ml full strength hypochlorite fluid (Milton) to 8 litres of cold water. The article must be immersed totally for a minimum of 1 hour before being rinsed and dried. Metal equipment should be autoclaved or, if large surfaces are involved, freshly activated glutaraldehyde (Cidex, Totacid) should be used.

To maintain standards of infection control, regular "in use" tests should be made by the bacteriology laboratory.

Quaternary ammonium compounds commonly and erroneously used as disinfecting agents are poor in action against coliform organisms, e.g. *Pseudomonas*, and are seriously inactivated by hard water and plastics. They are not to be recommended (Cetrimide, Savlon, Roccal, etc). They are of value only when it is necessary to cleanse wounds.

Staffing

The Senior Nurse

The nursing service provided for patients at their post-anaesthetic recovery time should be under the direction of one senior nurse. Her duties should be those of a departmental manager and a clinical nurse specialist. It is important that she should be readily available to advise and support her staff in clinical problems or procedures during working sessions.

She should have post-registration experience in anaesthesia and intensive therapy, in addition to having worked in operating theatres. Ideally she should have gained certification in one or more of these fields.

This nursing commission must primarily be the concern of the hospital's anaesthetic department and therefore the senior nurse will liaise with them to produce satisfactory policies and safe working standards.

The senior nurse should attend surgical ward divisional meetings in an advisory role. Amongst the important divisions with whom she should also have a close working relationship are the senior operating theatre nurse and her staff, the division of anaesthesia, surgical consultants and their ward staff, the district or hospital education division, the intensive therapy unit and the general hospital administrative staff.

The senior nurse should supervise the personnel of any part of the hospital which is undertaking a procedure which will include the giving of an anaesthetic. The ideal is for her to have her own mobile work-force. If this cannot be achieved then a training programme for every nurse caring for a patient after an anaesthetic should be implemented and the standard recovery equipment should be available at each site. Accident and Emergency, X-ray, Psychiatric, Maternity and Day Surgery Departments will all require this recovery training for their staff.

Staffing may include the usual grades of nurse but, being acute patient care, the auxiliary helper would best be employed in another area where her skills would be commensurate with her training.

In recruiting staff the aim must be to produce a well-planned in-service training for them. Previous surgical nursing and anaesthetic or ITU experience is a valuable adjunct and the offer of flexible working hours can produce useful recruitment of older nurses or those with family ties. With a positive approach to this teaching of recovery nursing care an enthusiastic team can be created, to the great benefit of the operating theatre unit as a whole.

Nurse–Patient Ratio

As safety is the keyword in patient care, it is right that there should be one nurse to one patient at all times. The post-anaesthetic period may not always produce a normal pattern in returning to a safe conscious level. A seemingly straight-forward progression through the reversing stages of an anaesthetic can some-times slow down or even regress. An apparently uncomplicated recovery can suddenly become a life-threatening crisis. The reasons may not always be predictable; to leave one patient's side to attend to the needs of another could well prejudice the zealous care needed by every patient throughout his recovery phase. It is only with hindsight that the patient's progress can be said to have been uneventful. A minor surgical procedure does not automatically preclude a difficult recovery time.

The fluctuating flow of patients to the recovery area causes problems in gauging the correct staffing levels. The shorter surgical operations of gynaeco-logical or ear, nose and throat lists will make for higher nursing staff require-ments. The end of a surgical list (which may also coincide with a meal-break) will need a bridging of staff duties.

The employment of recovery nurses during periods of comparative quiet is of no difficulty if they are directed to assess the progress of those patients currently in the operating theatres. Here they will be reviewing the anaesthetic technique being undertaken and the monitoring of the patient and be forewarned of any problems. They can also assist the operating staff when this is appropriate. It can be a time for instruction of junior staff or the planned teaching of students on secondment to the recovery area.

Twenty-four Hour Staffing

This nursing requirement is called for in the larger hospital where night emergency surgery is carried out. Staffing can be undertaken either on a rotational system to include a night-duty shift or with the establishment of a permanent recovery night staff. If one night-duty recovery nurse is to be included in the operating theatre team, then an allocation of four full-time staff members will be required to cover this. The alternative scheme of an "on call" rota is seldom satisfactory in practice. A nurse brought in for night emergency work would as a consequence deplete the staffing numbers for the following day.

Staff Training

To date there exists no national training syllabus for those nurses who wish to work exclusively in the post-anaesthetic recovery room. Standards at present vary from hospital to hospital. Individual recovery units have produced their own in-service training schedules but these are not recognised with a certification by outside examiners. A formal training course leading to the attainment of a certificate now exists in the USA. This should well be our goal in the UK but until this becomes a reality, an expansion of the ENB 182 course for anaesthetic nurses laying stress on recovery nursing skills should be a feasible alternative.

Those instructing new staff members or nurses gaining recovery room experience in their post-basic courses still have few books or resources to call upon at present. The specialty should be seen as an amalgam of the theories of anaesthesia, intensive therapy and surgical nursing. Clinical experience alone is not sufficient for post-anaesthetic recovery training.

Nurses in training gain by receiving lectures on the theory of the specialty before their secondment to the recovery areas. Their early practical experience must be recognised as possibly stressful for them. They will be exposed to the reality of surgical operations and the care of unconscious patients for the first time. Their allocation should be in working alongside an experienced and understanding member of staff while they gain in confidence.

It is certainly of benefit for nurses taking their post-basic courses in Accident & Emergency, ITU and Operating Department nursing to link their anaesthetic tuition with recovery experience. The programme will thus demonstrate the "cause and effect" of anaesthesia.

All recovery nurses must receive a thorough and frequently practised training in cardiopulmonary resuscitation, though the emphasis in our teaching is always to show how its need can be prevented by early supportive intervention. The skill of recognising and evaluating early changes in a patient's condition will be of the greatest importance to a nurse on her return to work on a surgical ward. She will be aware of the late effects of anaesthetic drugs on the patient and she will provide the needed continuity of post-anaesthetic care in the ward situation.

Nurse–Doctor Collaboration

The nurse receiving a patient from the operating theatre must be informed of relevant details of both the surgery and anaesthesia. This will mean that a good medical basis of understanding will be provided for the monitoring of the patient. Without the full picture of the patient's time in the operating theatre, she will have a far less interested and efficient approach to her nursing. The nurse will rely on the anaesthetist to pass on to her relevant information concerning the patient's operation and anaesthetic as well as particular instructions for the post-anaesthetic period (p. 24).

The full post-anaesthetic support of the patient will devolve on the recovery nurse and she undertakes this responsibility in working largely in the absence of the anaesthetist. His reliance on her will always be justified if he can be assured that all information on the progress of his patient will be swiftly conveyed to him (Chapter 4).

The patient continues to be the legal responsibility of the anaesthetist during the recovery period. That the nurse is caring for his patient does not absolve him in a court of law from his responsibility, though the standards of nursing care will also come under close scrutiny if problems occur. The record of the anaesthetic observations should continue into the recovery time. The patient's return to the ward should only be sanctioned by the anaesthetist or his deputy when these written observations have been reviewed and he has preferably seen the patient in the recovery unit.

This express permission given to the nurse should also hold good for his last patient on a surgical list. If the anaesthetist intended to leave the operating theatre unit before his patient's return to the ward, then the nurse would rightly need answers (which should be recorded) to the following questions:

1. Where may the anaesthetist be contacted?
2. How can he be contacted?
3. To which named member of the medical staff has he passed responsibilities for his patient should an emergency occur?

All post-operative orders should be given in writing by the anaesthetist or surgeon. The anaesthetist must be readily available to come to the assistance of the recovery staff. Outright emergencies may be prevented by early intervention, and if a nurse summons medical help quickly, she is to be congratulated for her alertness and never dismissed as having called him unnecessarily. She should never be given to understand that the action she took was other than conscientious recovery practice. If all goes well for 95% of patients it is still for the unpredictable 5% that she must be on her guard.

The anaesthetic responsibility for the recovery unit as a whole must be understood. With many medical users of the service it is desirable, though frequently not undertaken, to have a nominated anaesthetic consultant in charge of the department. An authoritative voice is needed to resolve both medical and clinical uncertainties. From experience, the balloon of an aired grievance seldom rises very high.

It is not often thought necessary for a duty anaesthetist to work solely in the recovery unit although a unit outside the confines of the operating theatre complex may warrant this allocation. An anaesthetist involved in intensive therapy work can be of assistance to colleagues if additional help is required for a short time with recovery patients. It presupposes a nearness of the two units for this to be a practical arrangement.

Policies of a Recovery Unit

It is sensible to lay down in writing the policies of a recovery unit. Systems of conducting this service vary from hospital to hospital and as yet it has not been standardised as it has been in the operating theatre itself. A written policy manual would define, for any one recovery unit, the pattern it should follow and would be a book of reference for all grades of medical and nursing personnel. Regular meetings involving all those concerned in the patient's recovery period should be arranged. It is then that policies can be discussed. If necessary, changes may be made and the manual upgraded. It is always important to include surgical ward representatives so that useful information can be exchanged.

Defined policies should include:

1. *The objects of the unit, namely:*
   a) Care of the patient through the reversing stages of anaesthesia
   b) Recording of observations on a recovery chart
   c) Treatment of complications of anaesthesia and surgery (Chapter 4)
   d) Transfer of the patient to the care of the ward staff once the criteria for discharge have been met (p. 51)

2. *Criteria for admission*
   Patients who have had diagnostic or surgical procedures following:
   a) General anaesthesia
   b) Local or regional anaesthesia
   c) Intravenous sedation
   d) Dissociative anaesthesia, e.g. ketamine
   e) Premedicant drugs
   Patients from dispersed recovery areas (e.g. day surgery units, angiography and radiography departments) who need further recovery care may also be admitted.

3. *The staffing grade* and responsibilities
4. *The minimum staffing levels per shift* to enable a ratio of one recovery nurse per patient to be maintained
5. *Health and safety regulations* pertaining to recovery work defined
6. *A list of available drugs*
7. *A post-anaesthetic training schedule*

In addition to these general policies, procedures must be laid down for the following circumstances:

1. *Patients detained in recovery unit* for prolonged periods or requiring transfer to the intensive care unit. Arrangements must be made for informing the ward staff and relevant medical personnel of the causative factors.
2. *Deaths occurring in the recovery unit.* A procedure agreed by the senior staffs of the recovery unit, the operating theatre and the ward should be carried out. Screening of a suitable area should be made possible. A full report of the circumstances leading up to the death should be recorded and given to the patient's ward as soon as possible. There should always be a sensitive approach in conveying the message.
3. *Patients bypassing the unit*
   a) Known infective patients, e.g. Hepatitis B carriers (HBV), Human Immunodeficiency Virus (HIV), and gas gangrene
   b) Patients destined for post-operative ITU care
   c) Patients returning to specialised units, e.g. neurosurgical or cardiothoracic units
   d) Patients whose surgery has been cancelled
4. *Night recovery work.* Patient care is similar to day procedures except that the patient will almost certainly be recovering from emergency surgery (see p. 111). Provision should be made for the patient's transfer either to his ward or to the ITU well before the start of the following day's surgical list.
5. *Major incidents/accidents.* The recovery service would be extended to give multipatient resuscitative care in this emergency, their skills being eminently suited to this.

Further Reading

Andrewes SJ (1977) Post-operative nursing in the theatre unit. NATNews April 14 (3): 10–18
Andrewes SJ (1984) The role and training of the post-anaesthetic PAR nurse. NATnews spec supp, Anaesthetic & post-anaesthetic nursing, Vol 21, No 7, July
Atkinson RS, Rushman CB, Lee J Alfred (1982) A synopsis of anaesthesia. 9th edn. Wright, Bristol
Clark MM (1973) Ketalar—a children's anaesthetic, Nursing Times, 69: 310–311
Codes of practice (1983) NATNurse, 3rd edn. 22 Mount Parade, Harrogate, UK
Dinsdale RCW (1985) Viral hepatitis, AIDS and dental treatment, Brit Dent J pub, London
Eltringham RJ (1979) Complications in the recovery room, J R Soc Med 72: 278–280
Farman JV (1978) The work of the recovery room. Br J Hosp Med 19: 606–616

Glenister HH (1988) Cross infection, aspects of HIV. J of Sterile Services Management, London, Vol 5, No 5, 15–17

Hollister GR, Burn JMB (1974) Side effects of ketamine in paediatric anaesthesia, Anesth Analg 53: 264–267

Howorth FH (1980) Air flow patterns in the operating theatre. Eng Med 9(2): 87–92

Howorth FH (1981) What's in the air of the operating theatre? NATNews 18: 17–19

Hudson RBS (1979) Pattern of work in the recovery room. J Roy Soc Med 72(4): 17–19

English National Board, 170 Tottenham Court Rd., London
    Course 100, General intensive care nursing
    Course 176, Operating department nursing
    Course 182, Anaesthetic nursing
    Course 183, Operating department and anaesthetic nursing

King Edward's Hospital Fund for London (1985), Re-use of sterile, single-use and disposable equipment in the N.H.S. Conference proceedings December 1985 London,

Lim-poh-choo v Camden & Islington Area Health Authority (1979) 3 WLR 44

Lunn IN, Mushin WW (1982) Mortality associated with anaesthesia, Nuffield Provincial Hosp. Trust, London

Macintosh R, Mushin WW, Epstein HG (1970) Physics for the anaesthetist. Chaps. XX–XXIII Blackwell Scientific, Oxford

Maurer IM (1983) Hospital Hygiene, 3rd edn. Edward Arnold, London

NATN (1987) Quality assurance tool 4, Recovery patient care. NATN with BUPA Hosps, Harrogate, UK

Post-anaesthetic recovery facilities (1985) Assoc Anaes GB & Ireland

Renfrew MJ, McManus R (1975) Recovery and reception area. NATNews 12(6): 13–15

Royal College of Nursing (1987) Introduction to HVB & nursing guidelines for infection control. Rcn Publications, London

Wakeley J (1974) Nuffield orthopaedic centre theatre complex. Nursing times 70: 1648–1650

Walton J, McLachlan G (eds) (1986) Partnership or prejudice, Nuffield Provincial Hosp Trust, London Department of Health and Social Security, London
    Antistatic precautions (1977) rubber, plastics & fabrics (011 320102 8)
    Antistatic precautions (1983) flooring in anaes areas (0 11 320680 1)
    Beren L (1969) Switches and socket-outlets in anaesthetising areas, DHSS letter Ref: G/H 39/6, 12th May
    Health Circular (1977) The extending role of the clinical nurse – legal implications and training requirements, HC(77)22
    Health Tech Memo No 82, (1983) Fire safety in health care premises, (0 11 320795 6)
    Hospital Building Note No. 26 (1975) Operating department
    Hospital Building Note No. 27 (1974) Intensive therapy unit
    Sharps disposable specification, TTS/5/330 015

Chapter 2
Normal Recovery

Physiology of the Elimination of Anaesthetic Gases

Patients recover from anaesthesia as the agents given to maintain anaesthesia are either excreted or metabolised.

Volatile agents are largely excreted unchanged by the lungs. However, a significant percentage of halothane (over 20%) is metabolised in the liver and then excreted in the urine. Lesser amounts of enflurane (2%) and insignificant amounts of isoflurane (0.2%) are also metabolised. Isoflurane is the least blood soluble of these three agents and halothane the most soluble. Theoretically, the less soluble an agent is, the faster should be the rate of recovery.

Suxamethonium is rapidly metabolised by pseudo-cholinesterase in the blood. Recovery from suxamethonium usually occurs within 3–5 minutes. Occasionally, a patient may lack pseudo-cholinesterase. Suxamethonium is then metabolised more slowly in the liver. This may take several hours. During that time, the patient should be ventilated and sedated. Subsequently, the patient's general practitioner should be informed and close relatives should be screened to determine if they too lack the relevant enzyme.

Non-depolarising muscle relaxants normally have their action reversed by an anti-cholinesterase (Neostigmine) at the end of the surgical procedure. However, two of the newer agents, atracurium and vecuronium, are short-acting and do not always need formal reversal. Vecuronium is metabolised in the liver whilst atracurium undergoes Hoffman degredation, i.e., it spontaneously breaks down at body temperature and pH.

Analgesics given pre-operatively or intra-operatively should preferably still be active so that patients do not recover consciousness to find themselves in severe pain.

To understand the reversal of an anaesthetic, when volatile gas agents have been used, is to recognise that the elimination pathway is similar to that of its uptake. The same physiological rules control the blood–gas partition coefficient and its solubility rating. At their withdrawal the anaesthetic gases, with their higher partial pressure in the venous blood carried by the pulmonary artery, diffuse across to the lower pressure of the alveolar space. A gas of low solubility in blood (e.g. nitrous oxide) will rapidly transfer to the alveolar space. The rate of fall of the alveolar concentration is in proportion to the patient's ventilatory performance.

We will therefore be seeing the importance of output controlled by blood: gas solubility, venous/alveolar partial pressure changes and cardiac and respiratory performance.

However, at the time of elimination, important factors adversely affect the smooth dispersal of the gases. The high concentrations of nitrous oxide which easily passed across the alveolar space have now displaced the oxygen of the inspired atmospheric air in the lungs. This is called *diffusion/hypoxaemia*, the Fink effect.

Cardiac output may well have become reduced by myocardial depression caused by anaesthetic drugs and respiratory function can be reduced by both hypercapnic and hypocapnic states if there exists any central depression of the brain's respiratory centre. This central depression may also obtain when major analgesic drugs have been used concurrently with the general anaesthetic.

First a yardstick should be established by which to assess the patient's normal progress at his post-anaesthetic recovery time. The variable effects of an anaesthetic will then more easily be noted.

Progress of Normal Recovery

Depth of anaesthesia is determined by physical signs and is classically divided into stages I–IV as described by Guedel.

During the recovery from anaesthesia the stages are seen in reverse order (Table 2.1).

Stage IV (medullary paralysis) is characterised by respiratory arrest and occurs as a result of an overdose of anaesthetic agents. This must be reversed at once and is not seen during the recovery period.

Stage III: Stage of surgical anaesthesia. During emergence from this stage, which is divided into four planes, there is a gradual return of muscle tone and reflexes (Table 2.2). The purely diaphragmatic breathing seen in the deeper planes is replaced by the normal pattern of breathing as intercostal tone returns.

Stage II: Stage of excitement. During this stage the patient may struggle and make unco-ordinated movements. Reflexes have returned and vomiting may occur. Difficulties may be encountered in extending a patient's forearm in taking a blood pressure at this time.

Stage I: Stage of analgesia. Analgesia is wearing off and the patient gradually regains consciousness. Female patients are liable to become tearful and male patients may be aggressive or amorous. Fortunately there is seldom any recollection of this.

Although progress of recovery may be assessed within this framework, it must be emphasised that many factors influence the return of consciousness, e.g. medical history, premedication and anaesthetic technique (see Chapter 6), so that a knowledge of these is essential for intelligent recovery nursing.

Table 2.1. Observations in the reversing stages of anaesthesia

Observations	Stage 3 Surgical anaesthesia	Stage 2 Excitement	Stage 1 Analgesia	Normal
Muscle tone		Tense or struggling		
Respirations (Intercostal / Diaphragmatic)				
Conscious level	Unconscious		Rousable	Conscious Cooperates Comprehends
Blood pressure, systolic		Fluctuating		Normal readings

Table 2.2. The returning reflexes

Reflexes	Stage 3 Surgical anaesthesia	Stage 2 Excitement	Stage 1 Analgesia	Normal
Swallowing Vomiting Laryngeal (cords) Coughing				
Bite reflex				
Eyelash reflex Eyelid reflex				
Secretion of tears				

Care Plan Nursing

The type of nursing required for the rapid turnover of high-dependency short-stay patients needs careful planning. No matter how many patients are seen nor how routine the procedure, each patient must be treated as an individual with particular needs. These needs will be related not only to the operation and the anaesthetic but also to a large extent to the patient's social and medical history. To nurse solely with information concerning the operative and anaesthetic procedure is to nurse the patient with some degree of ignorance. It is neither the time nor the place to be searching through the medical notes for information when the patient has already been admitted to the recovery unit.

To enable recovery staff to anticipate the patient's requirements, basic information should be available on each patient before his arrival from the operating theatre. It should be supplied either by the ward staff or, if it is practical, by the recovery staff following a pre-operative visit to the patient on his ward. This account of the patient will be recorded as a pre-operative picture of his needs and be transferred to the chart in the PAR room. Data processing facilities should if possible be made available for the unit.

The information required on each patient before operation should include:

1. Name and age, unit number (and marital status in the case of females) on identification band
2. Medical history of significance, with special reference to respiratory and cardiovascular systems with blood pressure and pulse rate
3. Drug therapy
4. Allergies
5. Skin state and general colour
6. Dental state
7. Hearing and vision problems
8. Command of English (a list of useful phrases in other languages can be found in Appendix B)
9. Emotional state
10. Belongings sent with patient, e.g. hearing aid, spectacles, toys
11. Weight
12. Haemoglobin and other biochemical results

The patient's identification wrist band must be checked for its accuracy. As well as the site of the proposed operation, the left or right side should be marked.

Reception of the Patient

When the patient arrives, the recovery nurse should, if possible, receive a full report from the operating theatre nurse. At the hand-over time of nurse to nurse, the report should include:

1. The patient's name
2. The surgical procedure performed
3. The name of the surgeon
4. The number and type of drains or catheters
5. The presence of packs remaining in situ

Inspection should be made of the wound dressing, the character and amounts of drainage and the diathermy plate site for evidence of burns. Instruction should be given by the surgeon regarding any special care to be exercised with his patient or any particular observations to be undertaken.

The anaesthetist will describe:

1. The anaesthetic technique used and its duration
2. The blood loss and intra-operative fluid replacement
3. The final monitoring record
4. Any complications encountered during anaesthesia
5. The post-anaesthetic requirements for
   a) the positioning of the patient   c) intravenous fluids
   b) oxygen therapy   d) drug therapy

Before the recovery nurse takes over the responsibility of the care of the patient she must satisfy herself on the following points:

1. His breathing is regular and unobstructed
2. He is maintaining a good colour
3. His pulse is palpable and regular

If she is concerned about any one of these vital considerations she should not hesitate to inform the anaesthetist while he is still at hand.

Basic Nursing Position and Safety

As with a tiny baby, the many needs of the unconscious patient should be anticipated. The nursing approach should be that of "positive protective care" and not just "tender loving care".

On arrival in the recovery unit:

1. The nurse should check that the patient is on the trolley the correct way round, i.e. so the patient can be tilted head down (Trendelenburg position)
2. She should station herself at the patient's head with all the necessary equipment within arm's reach
3. The brakes should be applied to the trolley or bed
4. The patient will normally be nursed on the side, and the position should be made secure with a supporting back pillow (see Fig. 2.1)
5. The side rails should be raised throughout the patient's recovery time

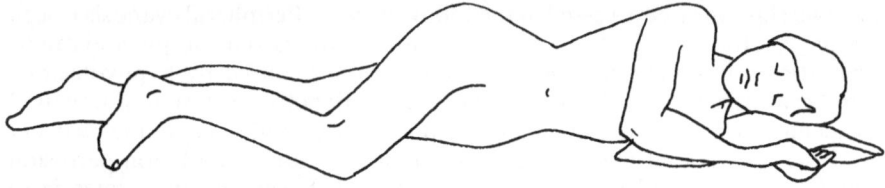

Fig. 2.1. Normal recovery position.

Routine Observations

As soon as the patient has been transferred to the care of the recovery nurse, she must assume full responsibility for the pateint's well-being until all the criteria for discharge have been met (see p. 51) and the patient is returned to the care of the ward staff.

The patient is kept under continuous observation and the findings recorded every 10 minutes. These recordings should not be seen in isolation but as part of a trend so that potential problems can be anticipated and corrected before a dangerous and possibly irreversible situation is allowed to develop.

The order of taking observations is as follows:

1. Colour
2. Respiratory function
3. Cardiovascular function
4. Level of consciousness
5. Blood loss

Following the baseline recordings on admission, an absolute minimum of three subsequent recordings are made at 10 minute intervals (i.e. for $\frac{1}{2}$ hour). If complications arise or if medications or units of blood are given, a further period of observation of at least 30 min will be required.

Assessment of Colour

With normal cardiovascular and respiratory function a supply of well-oxygenated blood is delivered to the tissues, which appear pink. If the blood is not being adequately oxygenated or the blood supply to the tissues is impaired, the normal pink appearance is replaced by cyanosis or pallor. If well-perfused areas such as the lips appear cyanosed, this indicates either respiratory or cardiac dysfunction and immediate attention must be given to these systems. In dark-skinned patients an examination of the inside of the mouth or the conjunctival vessels will provide the same information.

Peripheral and Central Cyanosis

These two signs may be assessed in the following way. Peripheral cyanosis is seen at the fingers, toes and tip of the nose. It signifies a low cardiac output and can be shown also in low systolic blood pressure readings caused by hypovolaemia. Central cyanosis, seen at the lips, tongue and conjunctiva, is a sign of impaired gas exchange between the alveoli and the pulmonary capillaries. In the recovery period the most usual cause is hypoventilation or lung ventilation/perfusion imbalance. A practical method to differentiate between the two states is to massage the cyanotic skin whereupon peripheral cyanosis will disappear, central cyanosis will not.

Assessment of Respiratory Function

Recovery staff must observe respiratory performance critically throughout the recovery period and recognise any departure from normal.

In normal breathing:

1. The patient's colour is satisfactory. There is no cyanosis of well-perfused areas.
2. The movement of warm expired air can be felt by placing the hand in front of the mouth or nose.
3. The chest and abdomen rise together with inspiration. The chest should not retract as the abdomen rises; this would produce a rocking or see-saw motion.
4. The breathing pattern is regular with a rate between 12 and 24 per minute in adults.
5. Breathing is silent. There should be no stertorous (snoring), stridor and no gurgling sound from the pharynx and there should be no wheezing.
6. Breathing appears effortless. The accessory muscles of respiration (sterno-mastoids and scalenes) should not be in use and the head should not retract with inspiration. The thyroid cartilage and upper trachea should not be drawn down during inspiration (tracheal tug). There should be no flaring of the nostrils on inspiration.

Any departure from the signs of normal breathing listed above must receive immediate attention since rapid deterioration in the patient's condition may follow (see Chapter. 4).

Assessment of Cardiovascular Function

When cardiovascular function is normal:

1. The tissues are well perfused
2. The pulses are easily palpable and regular
3. The heart rate and blood pressure approximate to normal pre-operative values

Tissue perfusion

Tissue perfusion is estimated by examination of the skin. This should be warm, pink and dry. There should be no pallor or cyanosis. Poor peripheral perfusion is indicated by cold pale extremities and a weak thready pulse. The nail beds provide a useful site for inspection. With variable lighting conditions a comparison of the attendant's own nail bed can serve as a useful reference. There should be a rapid return of colour following digital compression of the nail bed.

Pulse Measurement

The pulse may be taken at the following sites:

1. The radial artery at the wrist (in paediatric patients the brachial artery may be easier to feel)
2. The temporal artery (Fig. 2.2)
3. The facial artery as it crosses the border of the mandible in front of the insertion of the masseter muscle. This can conveniently be felt by the ring finger while maintaining the patient's airway (Fig. 2.3)
4. If these pulses cannot be felt, the carotid artery must be sought (Fig. 2.4) to confirm cardiac function

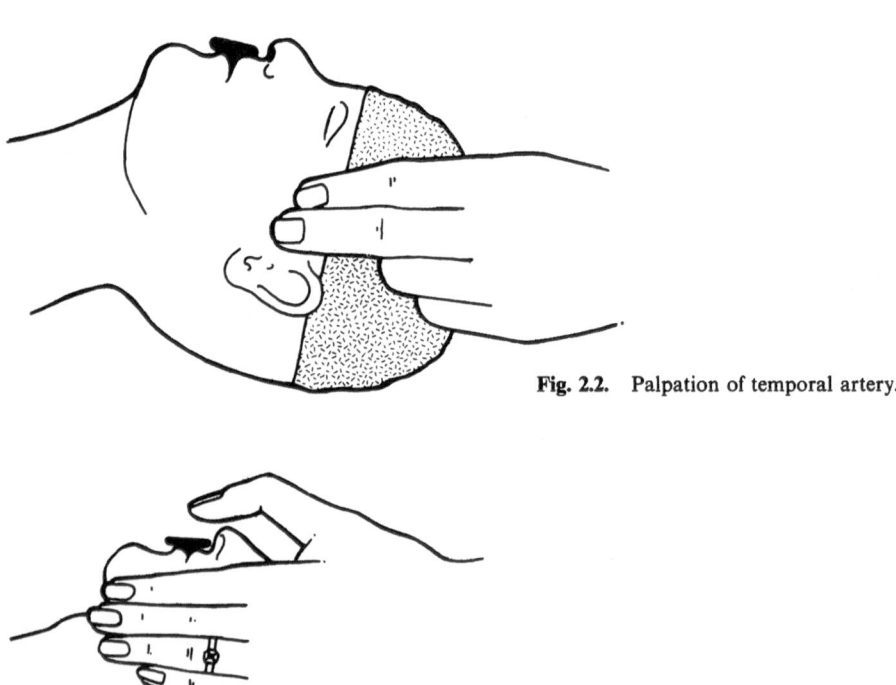

Fig. 2.2.   Palpation of temporal artery.

Fig. 2.3.   Palpation of facial artery with ring finger.

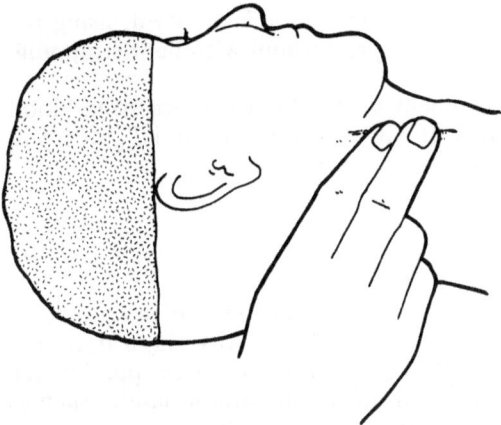

Fig. 2.4. Palpation of carotid artery medial and deep to the sternomastoid muscle.

In addition to the above, confirmation of the pulse at the following sites may be useful after vascular or orthopaedic surgery:

5. The femoral artery
6. The popliteal artery   } (see Fig. 2.5)
7. The dorsalis pedis artery
8. The posterior tibial artery

All pulse rates should be counted over a minute and any irregularities noted. If the pulse is weak and difficult to palpate, this should be recorded.

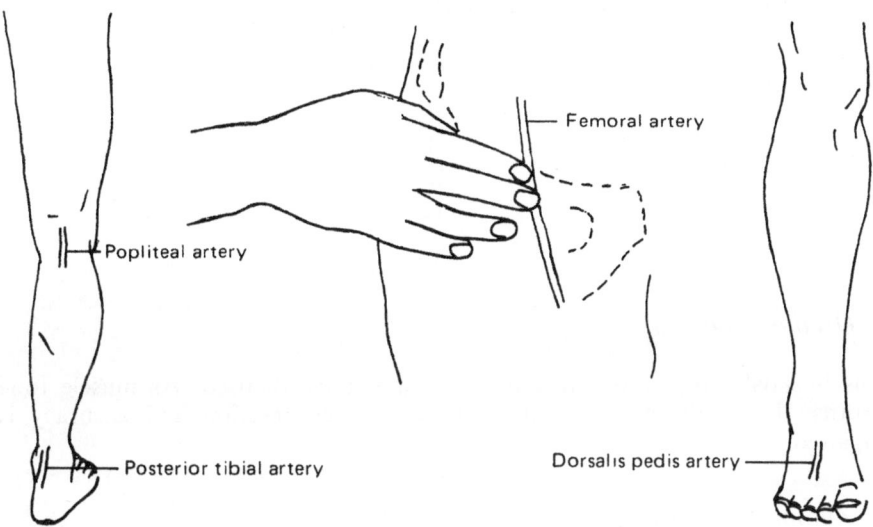

Fig. 2.5. Position of main arteries in the right leg.

With babies it may be more practical to listen to the heart itself, using the diaphragm of a stethoscope secured over the precordium with light strapping.

Doppler ultrasonic recorder. This instrument is of value when assessing blood flow when a pulse is not easily palpated. It will also confirm arterial patency in the limb distal to vascular surgical sites.

Blood Pressure Measurement

Absolute values of blood pressure are less important than a trend and should be interpreted in relation to the patient's general condition. Any major deviation from normal pre-operative values will require attention (see pp. 79–81), particularly if it is accompanied by other cardiovascular abnormalities such as poor peripheral perfusion or changes in heart rate or rhythm.

1. *Sphygmomanometer and Stethoscope*

It is important to use the correct size of cuff. With a standard cuff false high readings are obtained in the obese and false low readings in thin patients.

The width of the cuff bladder should be 20% greater than the arm's diameter (see Table 2.3). The cuff should be immediately deflated after use and removed if used on the same limb receiving an intravenous infusion.

Pulse pressure is the difference between systolic and diastolic blood pressure readings. A difference less than 40 mmHg may indicate falling cardiac output and therefore is a useful evaluation of the patient's perfusion state.

Table 2.3. Width of sphygmomanometer cuff bladder

	Bladder width (cm)	Length (cm)
Thigh	18.5	38.5
Obese	15	38
Adult	12.5	25
Child	8.5	18
Infant	6	12
Neonate	4	7.5

2. *Oscillotonometer*

This is satisfactory only when the patient is anaesthetised. As muscle tone returns, the needle swings with every muscle contraction and accuracy is impaired.

3. *Automatic Blood pressure Recording*

Various types of apparatus are available for automatic measurement and display of blood pressure using an oscillotonometer principle, e.g. the Dinamap,

Accutorr. Although these can save nursing time, they should not be regarded as an alternative to close observation of the patient.

4. *Direct Arterial Pressure Measurement*

During major surgery blood pressure is sometimes measured directly following insertion of a cannula into the lumen of an artery and the pressure displayed by an aneroid manometer (e.g. the Tycos manometer) or on a monitor screen via a transducer. Direct arterial pressure measurements are often continued post-operatively, and recovery staff should be familiar with the principles involved.

For accurate readings the transducer should be on the same level as the heart and must first be calibrated to zero at this level. To maintain the patency of the lumen the cannula must be flushed with heparinised saline either intermittently by a syringe or, preferably, by continuous infusion. This can be conveniently achieved by attaching a litre bag of sodium chloride 0.9% containing 1000 units of heparin via a giving set to the side arm of a continuous flushing device (e.g. the Intraflo). To maintain a slow infusion the heparinised saline is kept at a pressure of about 300 mmHg inside a pressure bag. If the arterial trace becomes damped or if a blood sample is taken from the arterial line it should be flushed with an additional bolus of heparinised saline.

The arterial cannula should be well away from intravenous infusion sites and must be clearly labelled as such, so that injections cannot inadvertently be given intra-arterially.

The cannulation site should not be hidden by dressings but should be protected by a small transparent covering to allow frequent inspection. This is necessary:

a) To detect impairment of the circulation occurring distally
b) To detect haematoma formation
c) Because disconnection will lead to severe blood loss

In the event of a) or b) occurring, or if measurements are no longer required, the cannula is removed. This is done using an aseptic technique followed by application of firm digital pressure via a sterile dressing on the cannulation site for a full 5 minutes. If bleeding continues after this, pressure must be maintained until it has stopped.

Additional information on cardiovascular function can be obtained by the following:

1. *Examination of venous filling*
The veins should be well filled and neither collapsed nor over-distended. Veins on the forearms and hand are suitable for examination. Neck veins are less useful in the supine position as they are generally distended unless there is severe hypovolaemia.

2. *ECG monitoring*
The ECG monitor records electrical activity of the heart but yields no information about its mechanical efficiency. It is not required routinely on all patients in the recovery room but can provide useful information on the nature of cardiac irregularities (p. 87) or evidence of myocardial ischaemia (p. 147). Its

use is recommended when there is a history of dysrhythmias or when pre- or intra-operative medications have been used to treat cardiovascular instability. Recovery staff should be able to recognise a normal trace and the common dysrhythmias and should refer abnormalities for interpretation, especially if accompanied by other evidence of cardiovascular dysfunction.

A full 12-lead record will be required if myocardial infarction or pulmonary embolus are suspected.

3. *Central venous pressure (CVP)*

This reflects a balance between cardiac output and circulating blood volume and can be measured by placing the tip of a catheter in the superior vena cava, the exact position being confirmed radiologically. Readings are taken by a simple manometer consisting of a column of fluid connected to an intravenous infusion by a three-way tap (Fig. 2.6), the meniscus fluctuating in time with respirations. Readings may also be taken via a transducer as for arterial pressure readings.

It is important that all readings are taken from the same well-defined anatomical landmark, such as the fourth thoracic interspace in the mid-axillary line. The normal range is 5–15 cm of water although absolute values are of less importance than the trend in response to therapy. In general, high readings suggest fluid overload or cardiac dysfunction while low readings suggest a reduced circulating blood volume.

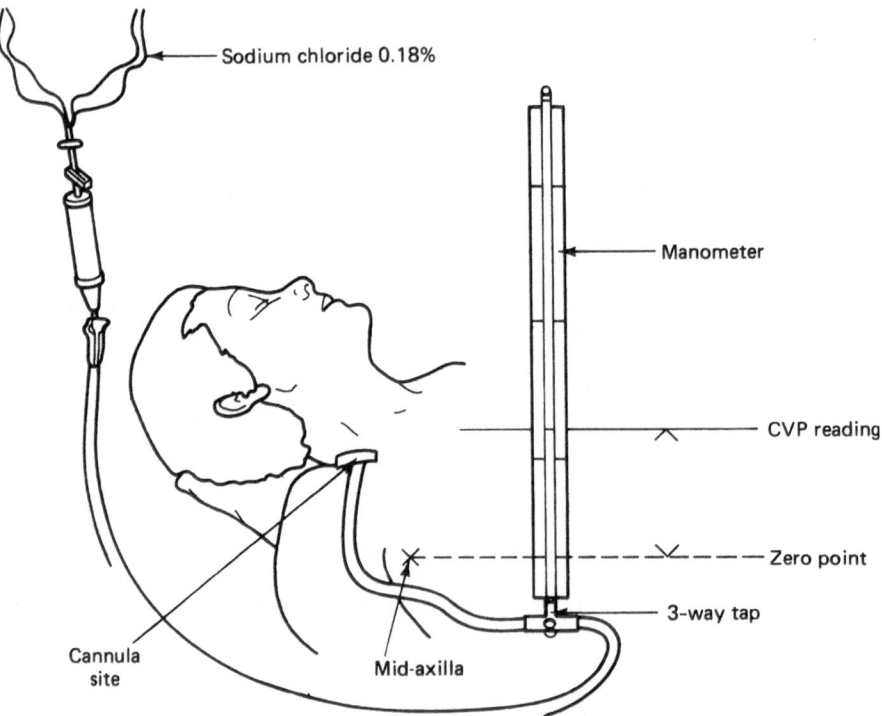

Fig. 2.6. Measurement of central venous pressure.

4. *Pulmonary capillary wedge pressure (PCWP)*

In the critically ill patient a discrepancy may exist between left and right ventricular performance. An indication of left ventricular function can be obtained by use of a balloon-tipped flotation catheter, e.g. the Swan-Ganz catheter.

The simplest type has two lumens; one measures the pressure at the tip and is connected to a pressure transducer, while the other is used to inflate the balloon with air. The catheter is inserted via a central vein into the right atrium, the balloon inflated with a maximum of 2 ml air and the catheter advanced until it wedges in the pulmonary artery. With the balloon inflated the pulmonary capillary wedge pressure is obtained. This reflects left atrial pressure. With the balloon deflated the pulmonary artery pressure is obtained. More sophisticated modifications may also have a proximal lumen opening into the right atrium and a thermistor at the tip for measurements of cardiac output by a thermodilution technique.

When a patient with a Swan-Ganz catheter in situ arrives in the recovery room, the transducer is re-calibrated, the pressure displayed on a monitor screen and the patency of the lumen maintained by a continuous flushing device as described under direct arterial pressure measurement (p. 31).

The recovery staff must be able to:

a) Identify the various lumens of the catheter
b) Recognise the pulmonary artery trace on the monitor screen
c) Inflate the balloon with air, identify the wedge trace and record the pressure
d) Deflate the balloon when this measurement has been made and ensure the pulmonary artery trace reappears

Care must be taken to ensure that the balloon is kept deflated between wedge pressure measurements, since prolonged wedging will cause pulmonary damage. The catheter tip may spontaneously advance into the wedge position, in which case it must be withdrawn until the pulmonary artery trace reappears.

Only sufficient air to produce a wedge tracing is required when inflating the balloon using a maximum of 2 ml. Over-inflation will cause pulmonary damage and may rupture the balloon.

If recovery staff are asked to remove the catheter it is important that the balloon is, of course, deflated first to avoid damage to the valves of the heart.

5. *Urine output*

Urine output is taken as an index of tissue perfusion in patients with healthy kidneys. An output in excess of $0.5 \, ml/(kg \cdot h)$ indicates adequate renal perfusion, i.e. 15 ml for a 60 kg patient every half hour. It is measured in a urine bag following the insertion of a Foley catheter. The bag is emptied and the amount recorded on admitting the patient to the recovery unit. Thereafter measurements should be made every 30 minutes. The presence of blood in the urine should be noted and the surgeon informed. Small amounts of urine cannot be measured with any accuracy using the graduations of a 1- or 2-litre bag. Drainage systems incorporating small volume urine-meters should be used or readings taken using a 50 ml syringe. The standard tubing from catheter to bag contains 3.5 ml per 10 cm length.

Assessment of Level of Consciousness

As soon as the anaesthetic administration ceases there should be a progressive return of consciousness as the agents are eliminated or metabolised. The level of consciousness is monitored:

1. To ensure that there is steady progress towards full consciousness and that there is no undue prolongation of unconsciousnes requiring investigation or treatment.
2. To determine when the patient has regained full consciousness, his protective reflexes have returned and he is able to maintain his own airway.

Elaborate monitoring as used following cerebral trauma is not required. The level of consciousness can be simply estimated by the following:

1. Return of eyelid reflex
2. Return of bite reflex
3. Response to moderate stimulation, e.g. gently rubbing the cheek
4. Ability to obey simple commands, e.g. "open your eyes"
5. Ability to respond to questions, e.g. "have you any pain?"

Hearing is one of the first senses to return following anaesthesia and can be demonstrated by an appropriate response to a simple question such as "Are you in pain?" or "Can you breathe easily?" Discussion of the patient's operative procedure or prognosis with colleagues should obviously be avoided. The above simple commands enable the patient to demonstrate his return to consciousness and ability to co-operate.

Painful stimulation is not required during routine recovery and should, as a practice, certainly be discouraged. It may be unpleasant for the patient, it may cause bruising and occasionally it provokes a violent response. Nevertheless, such stimulation may be used with discretion as a guide to progress if unconsciousness is unduly prolonged and a coma level assessment is required (p. 126).

Observation of the pupils is not routinely used as a guide to progress since many factors affect pupil size. When the anaesthetic agents have been eliminated, normal pupils are equal in size and react to light. Regular examination of the pupils is required after a period of cerebral hypoxia, following neurosurgery or cerebral trauma or if unconsciousness is prolonged.

Dilatation of the pupils (mydriasis) can be caused by:

1. Ganglion-blocking agents used to produce hypotensive anaesthesia
2. Large doses of atropine
3. Ether and cyclopropane administration and deep planes of anaesthesia
4. Mydriatic eye drops, e.g. cyclopentolate, phenylephrine

Constricted pupils (miosis) can be caused by:

1. Opiate administration
2. Miotic eye drops, e.g. pilocarpine

Recognition of Blood Loss

The patient may continue to lose blood in the post-operative period and evidence of this must be sought by regular inspection of wound dressings, packs, vaginal pad, drainage bottles and bladder irrigation. Continued bleeding must be referred to the surgeon and anaesthetist as further surgery and blood transfusion may be required.

If signs of hypovolaemia develop (hypotension, tachycardia, pallor or sweating) when there is no visible blood loss, internal haemorrhage must be suspected. The patient's girth measurements are seldom helpful as it is now recognised that internal haemorrhage can be extensive without an increase in the abdominal size.

Maintenance of the Airway

In the unconscious patient with the chin relaxed, the tongue is liable to fall back and obstruct the airway. To avoid this the head must be extended and the mandible held forwards. This can usually be achieved with one hand. The tips of the fingers are placed under the point of the jaw, which is lifted forwards and upwards so that the expired air can be felt against the palm of the hand (Fig. 2.7).

In the overweight patient with a short thick neck it may be impossible to displace the mandible in this way and a two-handed approach is required. The middle fingers of both hands are placed behind the angles of the mandible, which is lifted forwards. The fingers are spread with the forefingers at the tip of the chin, leaving the thumbs to feel the expired air or to hold a face mask (Fig. 2.8).

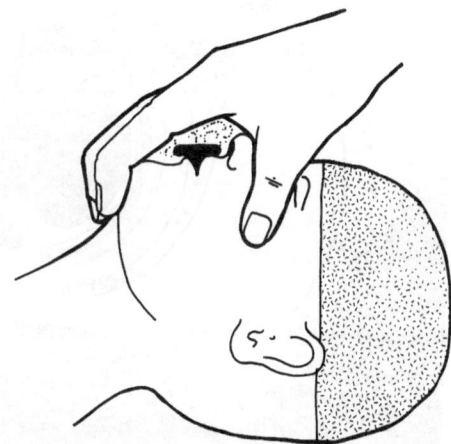

Fig. 2.7. Single-handed support of airway.

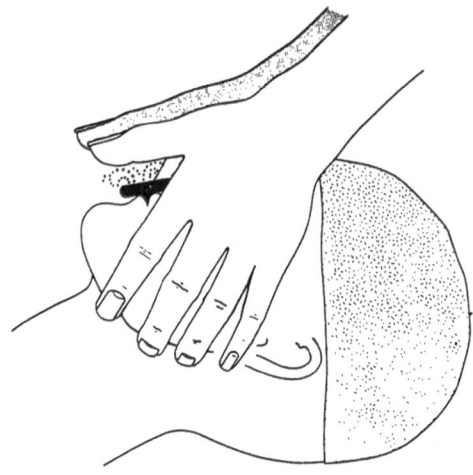

Fig. 2.8. Two-handed support of airway.

Insertion of Oropharyngeal Airway

An oropharyngeal airway, e.g. the Guedel airway, is inserted to prevent the tongue falling back thus obstructing breathing. Such airways are made of moulded rubber or plastic and come in various sizes:

Large males	Size 4
Standard adult males	Size 3
Adult females	Size 2
Paediatric range	Size 1, 0, 00 and 000

The size should be large enough to go beyond the back of the tongue but should not press on the posterior pharyngeal wall as this may stimulate the gag reflex. A

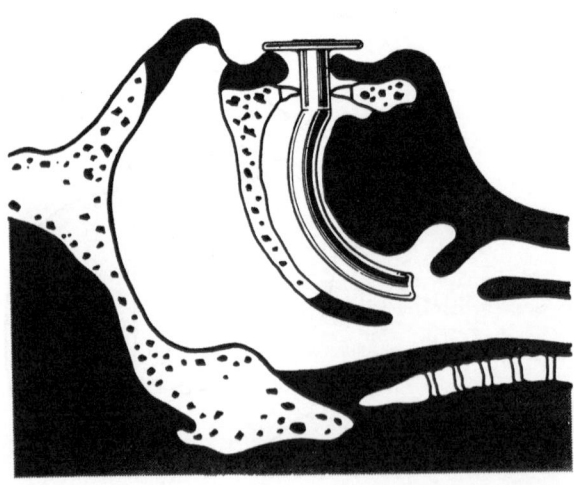

Fig. 2.9. Position of oropharyngeal airway (modified from diagram by Portex Ltd.)

check should be made that the rubber is in good order and that the metal insert is in place.

The airway is first lubricated with gel then introduced upside down and rotated in the vault of the mouth so that it slips down behind the tongue (Fig. 2.9). The patient's teeth (or gums in an edentulous patient) should bite down on the metal insert (flanged) end. Patency may be obliterated if the bite takes place on an unreinforced area. It should be checked that the lips do not come between the teeth and the airway as bleeding or swelling may result. It should also be checked that the lips do not fold over to obstruct air entry.

Insertion of Nasopharyngeal Airway

This may be required if:

1. The airway cannot be maintained using a Guedel airway
2. The jaws are clamped tightly together and it is impossible to insert a Guedel airway
3. The jaws are wired together following dental or faciomaxillary surgery (see p. 123)
4. Dental bridges and crowned or broken teeth are vulnerable to biting on a Guedel airway
5. There has been plastic surgery to the mouth

The nasopharyngeal airway consists of a curved tube with a flanged lip at the nasal opening (Fig. 2.10). It is manufactured to resist kinking and comes in four sizes of internal diameter, 9.0 mm, 8.0 mm, 7.0 mm and 6.0 mm.

To introduce the nasopharyngeal airway it is first lubricated and then inserted with half-rotating movements for its total length. Deviation of the nasal septum may indicate one side for easier insertion. Bleeding may be provoked and a fine suction catheter should be available which will fit inside the tube to clear the pharynx of blood. The introduction of a nasopharyngeal airway is unwise in patients on anticoagulants or with a bleeding disorder.

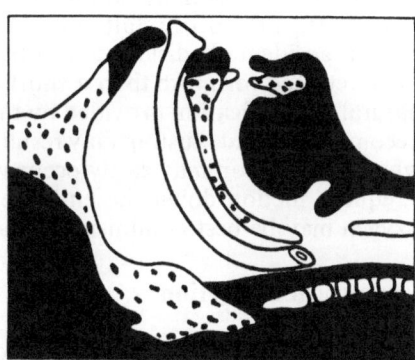

Fig. 2.10.   Position of naso-pharyngeal airway.

Suction of Upper Airway

Any fluid or foreign material in the mouth or pharynx should be removed by suction as it may:

1. Obstruct the airway
2. Irritate the larynx and cause laryngeal spasm during light stages of anaesthesia
3. Be inhaled into the lungs if the laryngeal reflexes have not yet returned
4. Provoke violent coughing spasms

The negative pressure (vacuum) setting, should be between 100 and 120 mmHg so that there is no damage to mucosal surfaces. Suction is indicated if gurgling sounds are heard during respiration, if the airway is obstructed and if there is breath holding or vomiting (see p. 95). Suction can be applied by a rigid Yankauer sucker or by a soft catheter. Catheter sizes range from F.G. (French gauge) 6 for neonates up to F.G. 22. The tip of the catheter can be advanced blindly behind the back of the tongue either beside or through the oropharyngeal airway. A catheter size F.G. 10 may be introduced down a Guedel airway.

After oral or throat surgery, suction should be performed by the anaesthetist under direct vision using a laryngoscope. Blind suction is inadvisable under these circumstances as it may dislodge clots or ligatures. A bowl of water should be available to clear the sucker if it becomes blocked by viscid secretions.

In susceptible patients suction may provoke bradycardia due to vagal stimulation. It may be noted that atropine given at the reversal stage of non-depolarising muscle relaxants will produce tenacious secretions affecting the respiratory tract. Unpleasant dryness of the mouth may be relieved, when the patient is fully arousable, by moistening the mouth with water on a swab. The swab should be mounted on a sponge-holding forceps.

Care of the Intubated Patient

Patients are occasionally admitted to the recovery room with an endotracheal tube in place. Recovery staff must be certain that it is well secured and does not become accidentally dislodged or obstructed by secretions or by kinking. If it is to be retained for more than a short period, humidification will be required as natural humidification provided by the upper airway is bypassed, secretions will become viscid and crusting may result. This is especially important in children in whom obstruction may easily occur with the narrower endotracheal tube sizes. Frequent suction down the entire length of the tube is required. Humidified oxygen may be best administered via a T-piece system (p. 42).

Endotracheal Suction

Before commencing suction, 100% oxygen is administered and the patient is warned of the procedure even if he does not appear to be conscious. A soft

Aeroflo catheter with an occluding port is used and the suction is set at 100 to 120 mmHg of vacuum to reduce mucosal damage. The nurse carrying out the procedure wears gloves for her own protection and handles the catheter with sterile forceps to avoid introducing infection. She passes the catheter down the endotracheal tube, ensuring the tip goes beyond the end of the tube; she then places her finger on the occluding port and slowly withdraws the catheter using a rotating movement, after which the oxygen supply is reconnected. The duration of suction should be limited to 5 seconds. This procedure is repeated using a fresh catheter each time until the trachea is clear.

Extubation

Before extubation is attempted:

1. Adequate spontaneous breathing must be established
2. Laryngeal and pharyngeal reflexes must be present
3. 100% oxygen is administered for several minutes
4. The larynx and pharynx are cleared by suction above the inflated balloon cuff
5. The tape or strapping securing the tube is released
6. The patient is on his side and head down if there is a risk of vomiting or regurgitation

An oropharyngeal airway (Guedel) is inserted, the endotracheal tube cuff is deflated and the tube removed at the end of an inspiration. The patient must be watched closely in the period immediately following extubation as respiratory difficulties are liable to occur at this time. Of particular importance are laryngeal stridor and laryngeal spasm, which will require immediate attention (p. 68).

The Ventilated Patient

If adequate spontaneous respiration is not established at the conclusion of surgery, the patient will require a period of controlled ventilation in the recovery room. Although many different types of mechanical ventilator are available, recovery staff must be familiar with the operation of the one in use in their unit.

The ventilator controls and gas flows are set by the anaesthetist but the recovery staff must know how to convert to manual ventilation should mechanical ventilation become unsatisfactory.

They may be required to monitor:

1. The respiratory rate
2. The tidal volume (which can be read from a Wright spirometer placed on the expiratory limb of the ventilator tubing)
3. The minute volume (tidal volume × respiratory rate)
4. The airway pressure. This is the pressure required to inflate the lungs. It usually falls to zero during expiration unless positive end expiratory pressure (PEEP) is added

5. The percentage of oxygen being delivered (an oxygen meter may be inserted into the gas supply)

Regardless of the type of ventilator in use and the settings on the dials, the chest must be seen to be expanding during inspiration and the patient's colour maintained. The ventilator may become disconnected or accidentally switched off and a ventilator alarm is advisable to alert nursing staff if this happens.

The anaesthetist must be informed immediately if:

1. The patient's colour deteriorates
2. The patient begins to resist the ventilator
3. The airway pressures alter
4. There are major fluctuations in the pulse or blood pressure

Oxygen Therapy

The supply of oxygen to the tissues depends on three factors:

1. The delivery of oxygen to the blood stream by a normally functioning respiratory system
2. The uptake of oxygen by adequate amounts of normal haemoglobin
3. The transport of oxygenated haemoglobin to the tissues by the cardiovascular system

Even young fit patients who have received a brief anaesthetic may benefit from oxygen therapy in the recovery period since all general anaesthetics can depress respiration. In addition, if nitrous oxide has been used, it dilutes the oxygen in the alveoli as it comes out of solution in the first few minutes after its administration (Fink effect). Following prolonged anaesthesia, a period of 30 minutes oxygen therapy will usually be sufficient to reduce hypoxaemia while the major depressant effects of anaesthesia are being eliminated (Meikeljohn 1987).

Additional indications of oxygen therapy in the post-anaesthetic period include:

1. *Any abnormality of respiration*
   poor respiratory effort
   lung disease (in the case of chronic bronchitis, see p. 146)
   reduced diaphragmatic movement following high abdominal incision and in the obese
2. *Reduced or abnormal haemoglobin*
   iron deficiency anaemia
   following severe haemorrhage
   sickle cell disease
   renal failure
3. *Abnormal cardiovascular system*
   cardiac failure
   myocardial ischaemia

4. *When oxygen requirements are increased*
    shivering
    thyrotoxicosis
    hyperpyrexia
5. *Restlessness and confusion*
    may signify cerebral hypoxia
6. *Whenever cyanosis is observed*
7. *When a blood transfusion is in progress*

Administration of Oxygen

Oxygen may come from a central piped supply or from cylinders, in which case spares must always be available. Ball and tube flowmeters are generally used, the base of the ball giving the correct reading. Where rotameters are used, readings are taken from the top of the bobbin, which must be seen to be rotating.

Oxygen masks should cover the nose and mouth, be well fitting and made of a clear plastic or vinyl material so that the colour of the lips can be reviewed. Although many different methods are available for oxygen delivery, two are commonly used in recovery units:

1. *A simple plastic moulded face mask,* e.g. Mary Catterall mask (M.C. mask Fig. 2.11). This is a variable performance type of mask, the inspired oxygen concentration (F_1O_2) varying with the flow rate and the patient's minute volume. At flows of 6 litres per minute an inspired oxygen concentration of 60% can be achieved. At low flow rates rebreathing may occur.
2. *Venturi mask.* A supply of oxygen enriches entrained air by the Venturi principle, known as high air flow oxygen enrichment (HAFOE) (Fig. 2.12).

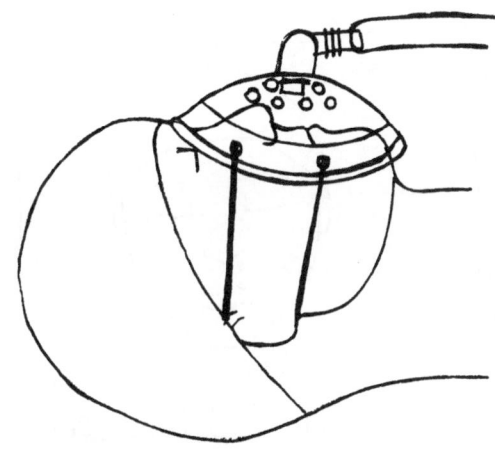

Fig. 2.11. M.C. mask.

The oxygen port is graduated to give a range of F_1O_2 between 24% and 36%. This type of mask is used when controlled oxygen concentrations are required, e.g. in patients with chronic bronchitis (see p. 146).

The patient should be told why he has a face mask in place lest he assume he is still being anaesthetised. If a face mask is not tolerated, the use of nasal cannulae can provide a suitable alternative.

For the patient who is intubated or has a tracheostomy, oxygen can be supplied via a T-piece system, the expiratory limb preventing dilution with air (Fig. 2.13). For the longer stay patient, the gases should be warmed and humidified.

If 100% oxygen is required, this can be provided using a closely fitting anaesthetic face mask and a Mapleson C circuit (Fig. 2.14). With spontaneous

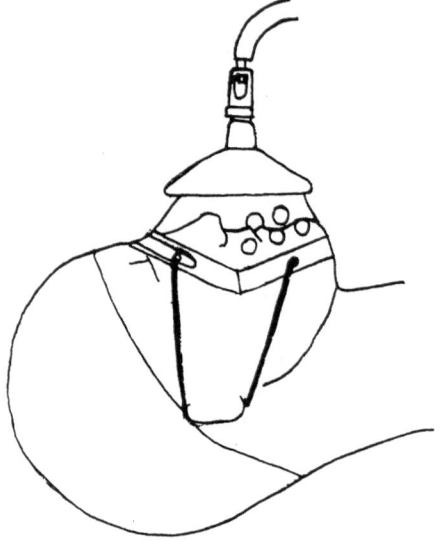

Fig. 2.12.   Venturi mask.

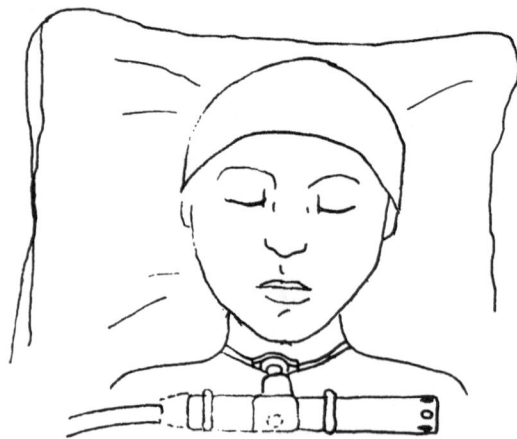

Fig. 2.13.   Delivery of oxygen via a T-piece system.

Heidbrink valve

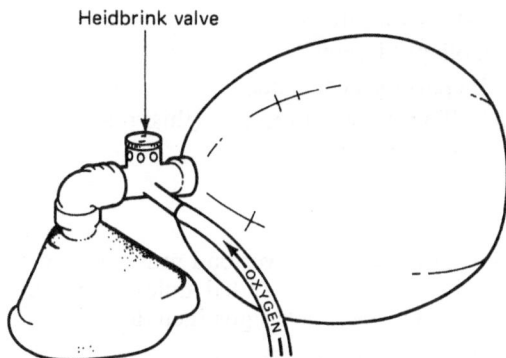

Fig. 2.14. Mapleson C circuit
with face mask.

breathing the Heidbrink valve is fully open to minimise expiratory resistance. With controlled ventilation the valve is partially closed to allow pressure to be generated in the reservoir bag for inflation of the lungs.

Maintenance of Fluid Balance

Measurement of post-operative fluid balance is vitally important. Assessment of fluid balance over a 12 or 24 hour period will frequently commence in the recovery period, so that it is essential that accurate records of both input and output, including all drainage systems, are assessed from the time of admission.

During those operative procedures requiring intravenous fluid therapy many factors will have been taken into account when deciding on the replacement regime. These include:

1. The pre-operative condition of the patient, e.g. state of hydration, electrolyte results, haemoglobin concentration, cardiac function
2. The fasting period pre-operatively
3. The patient's and the ambient temperatures
4. Evaporation from exposed tissues during surgery
5. Blood loss during surgery and anticipated blood loss post-operatively
6. Renal function

Although the intravenous regime may have been prescribed to cover the anticipated requirements of the subsequent 24 hours, it may require review during the immediate post-operative period as dictated by changes in the patient's clinical condition. Recovery unit staff should refer at once to the anaesthetist for advice when such changes occur.

If signs of hypovolaemia develop, the infusion rate is increased and evidence of haemorrhage sought. The signs of hypovolaemia include:

1. Pallor
2. Weak thready pulse

3. Cold extremities
4. Collapsed veins
5. Increasing heart rate
6. Falling blood pressure (this may be a late sign due to compensatory vasoconstriction)
7. Oliguria
8. Thirst

Signs of circulatory overload must also be recognised as a dangerous situation which can be compounded unless fluids are restricted in patients with poor cardiac reserve. Such signs include:

1. Distended veins
2. Full bounding pulse
3. Increasing blood pressure
4. Tachycardia
5. Breathlessness

Intravenous Infusion Drip Rates

Table 2.4 indicates the drip rate required to infuse 500 ml of fluid in a given time using a standard giving set from which 1 ml of fluid is normally delivered by approximately 16–18 drops. (Using the Metriset with paediatric patients the calculation is simpler as 60 drops equal 1 ml. Therefore the number of drops per minute is the same as the number of millilitres per hour).

Table 2.4. Intravenous infusion drip rates

Duration of infusion (hours)	Drip rate drops/minute (approx)
8	18
6	24
4	36
3	48
2	72
1	144

Intravenous Fluid Therapy

The integrity of the body will always have been violated by venipuncture and venous cannulation. Due precautions must therefore be taken to maintain sterility before, during and at the completion of intravenous therapy.

This will include the use of :

1. Sterile techniques
2. Sterile apparatus
3. Sterile fluids
4. Sterile dressing

Intravenous Infusions

Personnel should first wash their hands and, though a sterile trolley is seldom required for setting up an intravenous infusion (IVI), the sterility of the equipment must be maintained by assuring that no connecting parts become contaminated at assembly. The site of the IVI should be cleansed with a spirit-based skin preparation and shaved if necessary. A sterile occlusive dressing with a securing tape both to cover and to anchor the cannula should be used. The administration set should be labelled and initialled, giving the time of starting and the date. If there are more than one infusion in progress, the labels should have an identifying code, e.g. A, B and C. Once prepared, an administration set should be disposed of if it is not used within 4 hours since setting up.

Intravenous Injections

These should preferably be given by medical staff. Only qualified nursing staff who have received the appropriate training and have the necessary authorisation may administer drugs intravenously through previously placed cannulae. Authorisation may last for 1 to 2 years.

In hospitals intravenous drugs may only be given in accordance with their special rules. These cover:

1. The different methods by which nurses may give drugs intravenously
2. The procedures to be followed in giving and recording drugs by each method
3. Those authorised to give drugs by each method
4. The rate at which each drug should be administered
5. The amount and type of fluid which should be used if a drug needs to be diluted
6. The type and amount of a drug that a nurse may give

Blood Transfusion

To minimise the resistance to flow due to the viscosity of the blood a large intravenous cannula, e.g. F.G. 14, should be used. Strict precautions must be observed to ensure that the correct blood is given as clerical errors and inadequate checking are responsible for the majority of incompatible transfusions. The vital checking procedure is as follows:

1. The patient's full name and hospital registration number must correspond to those on the blood unit label.
2. The blood group and Rhesus factor on the cross match form must correspond to the blood unit label. In the case of rare groups, special arrangements are occasionally made with the transfusion laboratory for the supply of compatible blood of a different group. It is acceptable to infuse Rhesus positive into a Rhesus negative male but Rhesus positive blood should *never* be given to a Rhesus negative woman of child-bearing potential.
3. The blood unit number must correspond with the patient's blood transfusion form.
4. The expiry date must not have passed. Checking must be assiduous and no discrepancy either in the spelling of the patient's name or in the legibility of letters or numbers should be accepted. Once the blood has been checked and confirmed as satisfactory, the transfusion form is signed beside the corresponding unit number, witnessed by an assistant, and the transfusion commenced. The time is noted.

The patient must be observed frequently at the commencement of each transfusion so that reactions can be identified without delay (see p. 101).

Blood should remain refrigerated until it is required. It should not be removed for more than 30 minutes before administration in order to avoid the risk of multiplication of any previous bacterial contamination.

When large volumes are given rapidly, closer observation is required as additional hazards may be encountered (p. 103), and the blood units should be warmed as transfused.

Microfilters are recommended for blood transfusions exceeding two units. (p. 104)

Drainage Systems

When recording fluid balance, all drainage systems should be included, the amount and character or colour of the fluid being described. The following are used in the recovery unit:

1. *Urine drainage* (see p. 33)
2. *Nasogastric tube drainage.* When a nasogastric tube is in situ, it should be aspirated early in an attempt to empty the stomach. Although this cannot be assured using a narrow gauge tube, it will however reduce intragastric pressure and make regurgitation less likely. It should then be left on open drainage with the drainage bag secured at a level lower than the patient's stomach. The tube should be secured at the nose and again over the forehead or at the temple. The integrity of the cardiac sphincter has been breached by the presence of the tube which, if blocked or kinked, will not prevent

·vomiting or regurgitation taking place around the tube. If the patient appears nauseated, suction should at once be applied to the tube. A record of the amount and nature of the fluid obtained should be made. It is inadvisable for a nasogastric tube to be introduced during the recovery phase as this can promote vomiting.

3. *T-tube drainage.* A T-tube is inserted at surgery when the common bile duct has been explored–choledochostomy. It provides a safety valve when oedema may obstruct the flow of bile through the sphincter of Oddi with a consequent possible leakage into the peritoneum. It is required, therefore, as an overflow, not for the total drainage of the bile. Large quantities would only be seen if a complete obstruction existed in the common bile duct and would even then not be seen until later in the ward. It is preferable *not* to secure the bag with a safety pin but with adhesive plaster. In restless patients the tube could be pulled from the wound (Allan 1977). It is important that the bag is level with the patient and not beneath the bed or trolley lest a syphon effect be created.

4. *Ileostomy and colostomy bags.* These require to be directed towards the feet and not across the patient's side as, when he is sitting upright, there will be a gravitational flow. An emission of faecal fluid is unlikely in the post-anaesthetic time but the stoma area should be observed for blood loss. The adhesive fit between the neck of the collecting apparatus and the skin must be maintained.

5. *Vacuum drainage bottles.* When the antennae on top of the bottle are pointing laterally the bottle is at a negative pressure and functioning correctly. If there is a loss of vaccum, i.e. with the antennae vertical, further suction can be applied to the bottle. A sterile rigid sucker end should be used. Further vacuum failure will require the advice of the surgeon. If no fluid drains along the tubing to the bottle, an inspection must be made at the site of entry to the tissues for evidence of swelling or haematoma. This might indicate that the proximal end of the tube is blocked. The surgeon should then be consulted.

6. *Bellow drains – low vacuum.* These compressible plastic containers must be checked for maintenance of vacuum. They are used for superficial tissue drainage. As there can be no graduated marks on this type of apparatus, the volumes they contain cannot be accurately measured but the amounts are usually small.

7. *Chest drainage* (see p. 128)

8. *Bladder irrigation* (see p. 132)

Record Keeping and Charting

For the understanding of the needs of any one patient, and to promote a skilled and intelligent approach to recovery nursing, the recovery unit will require a charting system designed for its special needs. One of its main functions, other than being an accurate record, is its use as a tool. Serial recordings will show improving or stable parameters or swiftly reveal trends which require immediate correction. An interpretation must be made and an understanding of the physiological signs is required. Anything less than this is to ignore the importance of this short-term vital charting. The chart should be of adequate size and have an identifiable colour. At the top of the chart there should be space for:

1. Patient identification
2. Relevant medical history
3. Drug therapy
4. Relevant pre-operative recordings, e.g. weight, blood pressure, heart rate and haemoglobin concentration

There should be space on the chart to record:

 1. Time of observation
 2. Colour
 3. Respiratory rate and depth
 4. Pulse rate and rhythm
 5. Blood pressure
 6. Level of consciousness
 7. Oxygen concentration administered
 8. Intravenous infusion
 9. Drug therapy
10. Operation site review
11. Recovery nurse's signature

A simple example is given in Fig. 2.15. The reverse side is available for continuation.

The information above the double line is completed pre-operatively in the anaesthetic room or reception area by the recovery staff and the chart is then sent to the recovery unit. It is there attached to a clipboard at the patient's bay to await his admission. The example shown allows for observations over a period of 1 h 40 min. As the average length of a patient's stay is 30–45 min, it covers a satisfactory time span in most cases.

A continuation of the anaesthetic record chart is used by some recovery units, marking their observations in red at the changeover. They are, however, ill-suited for recording the special observations necessary for the recovery service. This also applies to the design of the surgical ward chart. On the other hand, when a specific recovery room chart is used the ward staff can easily continue to record their observations on it, as it has all the features needed to review the patient's immediate post-operative state. The clinical signs are clear to read in sequence, any one line of observations showing an easy evaluation which relates to previous recordings.

If a patient requires ventilatory support in his recovery time, a special chart should be provided (Fig. 2.16).

The accurate recording of the patient's progress after a given anaesthetic is of great value should further surgery be required at a later date. It may also be of great import for medicolegal cases when the recovery charting and the staff carrying out patient care will come under close scrutiny.

POST-ANAESTHETIC RECOVERY AREA			
Date..................................			Theatre..................................
Full Name	Hosp. No.	Age	Ward
PRE-OPERATIVE MEDICAL HISTORY	Respiratory	Cardiovascular	Abnormal Signs
Drug Therapy	Allergies		Hb / B/P / P

Time 10 Mins.	R	Pulse R/I	Colour	B/P	O_2	Infusions–Drugs	General Observations, Conscious Level	Operation Site
						Recovery Nurse		

Fig. 2.15. Recovery room chart.

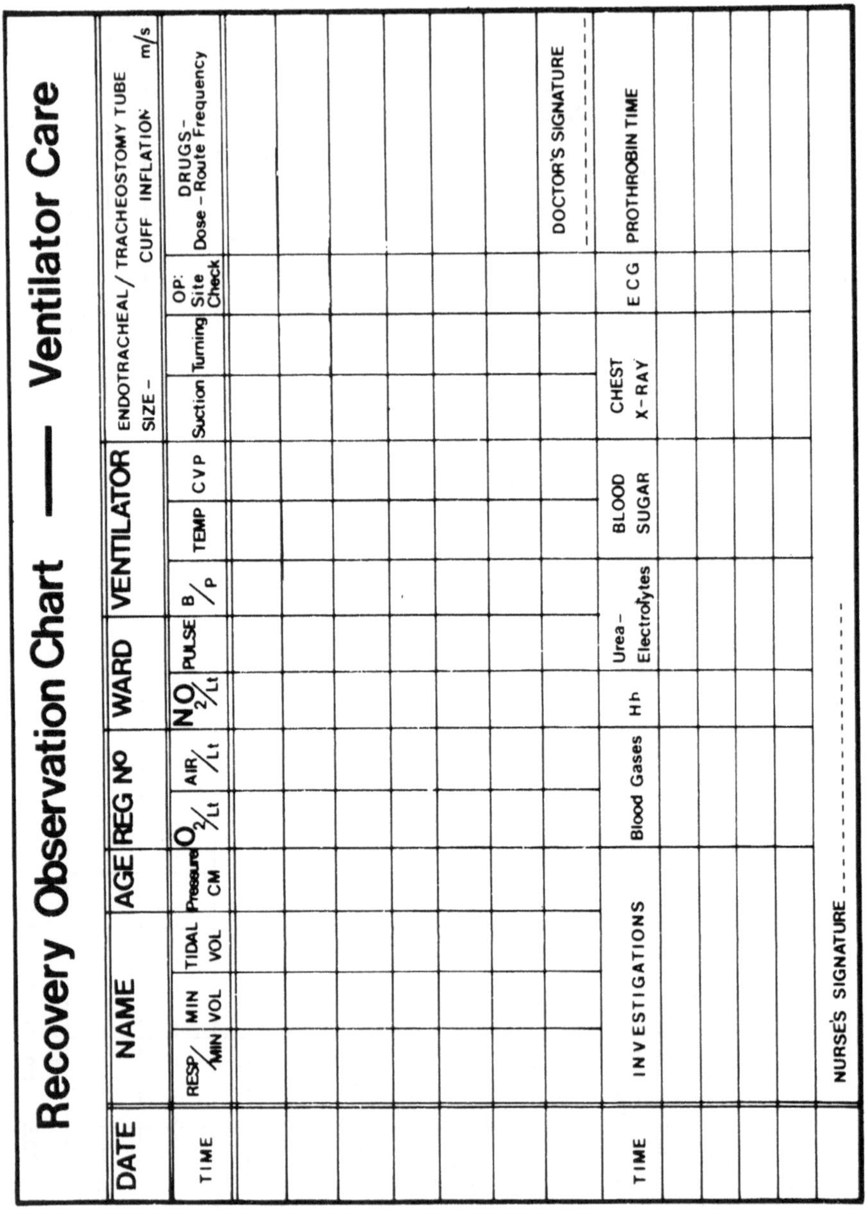

Recovery Observation Chart — Ventilator Care

DATE	NAME	AGE	REG No	WARD	**VENTILATOR**			ENDOTRACHEAL / TRACHEOSTOMY TUBE
								SIZE – CUFF INFLATION m/s

TIME	RESP/MIN	MIN VOL	TIDAL VOL	Pressure CM	O₂/Lt	AIR/Lt	N₂O/Lt	PULSE	B/P	TEMP	CVP	Suction	Turning	OP: Site Check	DRUGS – Dose – Route Frequency

DOCTOR'S SIGNATURE

TIME	INVESTIGATIONS	Blood Gases	Hb	Urea-Electrolytes	BLOOD SUGAR	CHEST X-RAY	E C G	PROTHROBIN TIME

NURSE'S SIGNATURE - - - - - - - - - - - -

Fig. 2.16. Recovery room chart for ventilated patients.

Criteria for Discharge

Discharge to a Ward

Before each patient is discharged to a ward the recovery staff must be satisfied that:

1. The patient is fully conscious, his reflexes have returned and he can protect his airway
2. Breathing is adequate and a good central colour is maintained
3. The cardiovascular system is stable. Consecutive readings of pulse and blood pressure approximate to normal pre-operative values, peripheral perfusion is good, and there is no unexplained cardiac irregularity and no persistent bleeding
4. The patient is comfortable, not in pain. Patients should remain in the recovery unit for 30 minutes following the administration of drugs to enable their effects to be observed. The assessment of blood transfusions also may delay a patient's return to the ward
5. Nerve blocks have receded. The patient is able to appreciate light touch and motor function has returned (p. 65).

Once the above criteria have been met, the patient and the linen are clean and the paperwork is complete, it is then safe to return the patient to the ward. Before contact with the ward is made, the discharge must first be sanctioned by the anaesthetist or by a deputy nominated by him.

Under no circumstances should a patient be discharged prematurely from a recovery area into the care of possibly less experienced staff on a ward. In the dimmed lighting of a ward at night, this may become an added problem. In hospitals with an emergency surgical service, recovery facilities must be available at all times (i.e. throughout the 24 hours and at weekends). In those hospitals that undertake little emergency surgery, the anaesthetist and operating theatre staff should monitor the patient's recovery until it is safe for him to return to his ward.

Failure to provide adequate nursing care for patient's during a period in which they are vulnerable and at risk of serious complications is unacceptable. Not only is the patient's life and well-being endangered but it may also prove extremely expensive for those responsible.

Once all the above criteria have been met and the patient's discharge has been approved by the anaesthetist or his deputy, he may be returned to the ward. He should be accompanied by a trained and experienced nurse.

Discharge to Intensive Care or High Dependency Unit

Should a patient's recovery from anaesthesia be prolonged or complicated, it may become necessary for him to be transferred to an intensive care or high dependency unit rather than return to a general surgical ward. It is obviously an advantage if these units are close to the main recovery area since transfer over a large distance can be hazardous. All patients should be adequately monitored during transfer. If transfer to a specialised unit is delayed, the recovery unit should be able to provide short-term intensive care including mechanical ventilation.

Transfer of Patient to Ward Staff

A trained member of the ward nursing staff or recovery room should escort the patient from the recovery unit. She should be given the following information (but not within the hearing of the patient):

1. The patient's name
2. The nature of the surgery performed
3. The names of the surgeon and the anaesthetist
4. The anaesthetic technique used, e.g. general, regional, hypotensive
5. The relevant information concerning drains, catheters, packs and suture materials
6. The progress of the patient in the recovery period
7. The post-operative requirements concerning oxygen therapy, position and frequency of observations

The anaesthetic record, the recovery room chart and the prescription sheet accompany the patient to the ward.

Further Reading

Allan D (1977) Complications of T tube drainage. Nursing Times Aug 1270–1271
Allen D (1988) Making sense of suction. Nursing Times Vol 84, No 10, 46–47
American Medical Association (1988) General Principles of blood transfusions. AMA, Monroe, Wisconsin, USA.
Andrewes SJ (1979) The recovery room as a nursing service. J R Soc Med 72 : 275–277
Beal JM (1966) Manual of recovery room care. Macmillan, New York
Belinkoff S (1967) Manual for the recovery room. Churchill Co. London
Betschman LI (1967) Handbook of recovery nursing. Davis, Philadelphia
Dale RF, Lindop MJ, Farman JV, Smith MF (1986) Autotransfusions, an experience of 76 cases. Annals Roy Col Surg Vol 68, 295–297
Evans FT, Gray TC (1965) General anaesthesia. 2nd edn. Vol 2, Butterworths, London
Farman JV (1973) Anaesthesia and the E.M.O.System. English Universities Press, London
Gray TC, Nunn JF (eds) (1971) general anaesthesia, 3rd edn. Vol 1, p, 449 Butterworths, London
Kember NF (1982) An introduction to computer application in medicine. Edward Arnold, London
Kinney JM, Bendixen HH, Powers SR (1977) Manual of surgical intensive care. WB Saunders, Philadelphia, London
Kirkendall MD, Burton AC, Epstein FM, Freis ED (1967) Recommendations for human blood pressure determinations by sphygmomanometers. American Heart Association
Levine A, Imai P (1983) Autotranfusions. American Operating Room Nurses, USA Vol 37/6, 1061–1064
Meikeljohn BH (1987) Arterial oxygen desaturation during post-operative transportation. Anaes Vol 42, !313–1315
Milne C (1988) Computers in nursing. Nursing Standard Vol 2/37 pp 32–33
Nicholson E (1988) Autologous blood transfusions Nursing Times Vol 84/2 33–35
Nunn JF (1969) Applied respiratory physiology. 282–283 Butterworths, London
Wallace CJ (1981) Anaesthetic nursing. Pitman Medical, London
Ward CS (1985) Anaesthetic equipment, 2nd edn. Baillière Tindall, London
Wilson R, Gaer J (1988) Right atrial electrocardiography in placement of central venous catheter. Lancet Vol 1, 462–463

Chapter 3

Pain Relief and Local Anaesthesia

Introduction

Most surgery causes pain and so there will be very few patients who do not require some form of analgesia post-operatively. The provision of adequate analgesia throughout the post-operative period is difficult and many patients suffer severe pain after their operation. This failure to provide proper pain relief has been rightly criticised as one of modern medicine's greatest failings.

Gate Control Theory of Pain

Formerly it was thought that pain was appreciated when specific peripheral receptors were stimulated and that sensation was then carried along pain fibres and pathways to a pain centre in the brain where it was perceived. This is no longer believed to be the case. Painful stimuli are transmitted along a variety of fibres ($A\beta$ and C) to cells in the dorsal horn of the spinal column where they synapse. The cells in the dorsal horn may either allow painful sensation to continue up the cord to the brain or, alternatively, they may prevent further onward transmission. This is the 'gate' proposed by Melzak and Wall (Fig. 3.1). If the gate is 'open', pain is felt; if it is 'closed', pain is not perceived. The gate can be closed either by further peripheral stimulation from $A\beta$ fibres or by inhibition by fibres descending in the spinal cord from the brain. Peripheral $A\beta$ fibres may be stimulated by friction (rubbing the pain away), the use of counter-irritants or muscle activity whilst central inhibition occurs naturally when an individual is concentrating intensely on other matters. A common example is the sportsman who does not notice injuries until after the game is over.

An ever-increasing number of transmitter substances are being identified as playing a part in either the appreciation of pain or in its inhibition. Much attention has recently centred on endorphin, the body's own morphine-like substance. Although it undoubtedly plays a role in pain control, it is only one among many such substances. As we discover more about how pain is transmit-

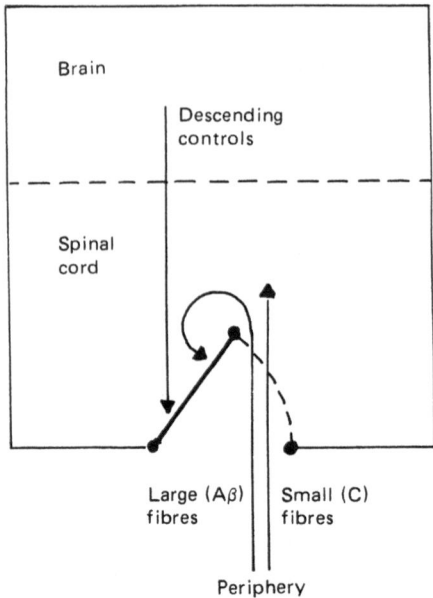

Fig. 3.1. Gate control of pain.

ted, we are better able to understand not only how narcotics work, but also how more esoteric forms of pain relief such as acupuncture, meditation and placebos exert their effects.

Although most patients expect some discomfort after surgery, no patient should be allowed to remain in pain in the recovery room nor be discharged back to their ward if their pain has not been relieved. The amount of pain relief required by any given patients will, however, vary and so each patient's needs must be assessed individually.

Factors that influence the amount of pain experienced post-operatively include:

1. The site of the operation
2. Analgesics given for premedication or used intra-operatively
3. The concomitant use of regional anaesthetic techniques
4. The patient's personality and state of mind

Any patient who says he is in pain should be believed even if the operation was 'trivial' and not usually associated with much post-operative pain. Similarly, patients may be in pain despite having received intra-operative narcotics or a nerve block. Additionally, staff should look for signs of inadequate analgesia in those patients who cannot adequately express their discomfort. These include:

1. Infants and children
2. Patients who are intubated or have a tracheostomy
3. The mentally handicapped
4. Patients whose native language is not English

Signs of inadequate pain relief may include:

1. Restlessness
2. Hypertension
3. Tachycardia
4. Sweating and lachrymation
5. Rapid shallow respiration

Methods of Pain Relief

Analgesic Drugs

Opiates remain the drugs most commonly used for post-operative analgesia. Most doctors have a preferred opiate but there is probably little to choose between them when they are used for acute pain. All the commonly used drugs (morphine, papaveretum, pethidine, etc) are equally effective providing adequate amounts are given. All have similar side-effects.

1. Respiratory depression
2. Nausea and vomiting
3. Hypotension
4. Alteration of mood and sedation
5. Pupillary constriction
6. Smooth muscle contraction leading to bronchoconstriction, biliary or renal colic and constipation

The first three listed are the most important in the recovery room. They should always be looked for in patients who have been given narcotics and, if found, treated immediately.

Should serious respiratory depression occur, it can be readily treated with intravenous naloxone. However, unless the dose is carefully titrated, naloxone will also reverse the analgesia. For this reason, many doctors prefer to first treat respiratory depression with doxapram which stimulates respiration but does not reverse analgesia. It should also be remembered that naloxone is a short-acting drug. It is possible for a patient treated with naloxone to suffer further respiratory depression after appearing to recover, particularly if they are continuing to absorb opiate from a bolus intramuscular injection.

Although nausea and vomiting are common side-effects of opiates, they do not inevitably occur. Anti-emetics should not be given routinely as they produce side-effects of their own but it is sensible to ensure that they are prescribed so that they can be given if indicated.

Although many opiates can be given orally or rectally as well as by injection, the intravenous route is to be preferred when rapid relief is required. Small increments of the chosen drug should be given and the effect monitored. There is no 'correct' or maximum dose. Increments should be repeated until the pain is relieved. If the patient appears to require an unusually large amount of drug the injection site should be carefully checked to ensure that the cannula is still in the vein. Other treatable causes of the patient's discomfort, such as a full bladder, should be excluded.

The intramuscular route, although widely used, is very much a second best choice. Absorption is slow and adequate analgesia may not be obtained for 30 min or more, especially if tissue perfusion is impaired. In addition, titration to the optimal dose is not possible so that either the pain may be inadequately relieved or the patient is over-sedated by a standard dose of narcotic.

Particular care is required when opiates are given to the following groups:

1. Patients with chronic airways disease
2. Patients taking monoamine oxidase inhibitors
3. Patients who have undergone neurosurgery or suffered a recent head injury
4. Children and elderly patients
5. Hypotensive patients

Opiates should not be withheld from the above groups; indeed a chronic bronchitic may breathe more easily and a head-injured patient may co-operate more fully with regular neurological assessments if their pain is adequately relieved. Likewise it is a myth that infants and the elderly feel less pain than other age groups. They should be given analgesia like all other patients but the optimal dose must be carefully assessed. It is also incorrect that addiction can be produced by over-generosity with post-operative analgesics. A patient with high post-operative analgesic requirements should not have his analgesia rationed any more than a diabetic with a high insulin requirement would have that rationed.

Partial Antagonists

Buprenorphine, meptazinol, nalbuphine and pentazocine differ from the other potent analgesics in that they have both agonist and antagonist properties and so can reverse the effects of other opiates and precipitate withdrawal symptoms in addicts. They are effective analgesics and are not subject to Schedule 2 of the Misuse of Drugs Regulations (UK) so no register has to be completed before they can be administered. However, they produce a similar spectrum of side-effects to the agonist opiates, with perhaps a higher incidence of hallucinations and dysphoria, and often show a ceiling effect in that, above a certain dose, further increments produce no more analgesia but only further side-effects. As the sequential use of agonists and antagonists can lead to a pharmacological muddle, their use in the recovery room is probably best avoided.

Patient Controlled Analgesia

A recent promising innovation has been the development of Patient Controlled Analgesia (PCA). A syringe of analgesic is connected to the patient's intravenous cannula. A slow infusion of analgesic is administered by a syringe driver and the patient can self-administer further boluses as and when they are required by pushing a button. The syringe driver contains micro-electronic circuitry that is pre-programmed with the infusion rate, the size of the boluses and the frequency with which they can be administered. Patients who have used PCA generally claim to have had better post-operative analgesia than patients treated by more conventional methods even though, on average, they have not given themselves more analgesic. The amount of drug administered by the patients to themselves, however, varies greatly, emphasising once again how much patients' drug requirements differ. Currently the high cost of the PCA apparatus limits its more widespread use.

Local Anaesthetic Techniques

After a period during which they were little used, local anaesthetic blocks are again gaining popularity, both as an alternative to general anaesthesia and for post-operative analgesia. Like every other technique they have their advantages and disadvantages.

Advantages:

1. No loss of protective reflexes
2. Little cardiovascular or respiratory depression
3. Good operating conditions with reduced blood loss, muscle relaxation and patient cooperation
4. Less systemic upset with reduced hangover-effect, less nausea or vomiting and a lower incidence of deep venous thrombosis
5. Smooth pain-free recovery

Disadvantages:

1. Time consuming to perform
2. Extra skill necessary to reliably perform the block
3. The consent and cooperation of the patient and surgeon is necessary
4. They are only useful for a limited range of operations
5. They are contra-indicated in the presence of clotting defects or sepsis at the site of skin puncture

but a local anaesthetic block can frequently, with advantage, be combined with a general anaesthetic.

Some of the problems and complications that can occur are common to all local anaesthetic procedures whilst others are specific to certain blocks. Complications may be either local, at or about the site of injection, or systemic.

Local complications include:

1. Infection
2. Ischaemia if adrenaline-containing solutions are used
3. Haematoma
4. Nerve damage
5. Damage to other local structures e.g. pneumothorax

Systemic complications. These are usually due to either an excessively large dose of local anaesthetic being given or an appropriate dose being absorbed too rapidly or being inadvertently injected into a blood vessel. They may be:

Neurological: restlessness, tremor, convulsions, medullary depression leading to respiratory and cardiac failure.

Cardiovascular: tachycardia and hypertension (if adrenaline-containing solutions are used), myocardial depression with bradycardia and hypotension if plain solutions are used.

Psychogenic: bradycardia and hypotension leading to fainting can be vagally mediated in nervous patients or those with a fear of needles.

Management of Toxic Reactions

As always, prevention is better than cure. The frequency of toxic reactions can be reduced by:

Not exceeding the recommended maximum dose of the local anaesthetic being used

Maintaining verbal contact with the patient whilst the block is being performed

Aspirating frequently whilst the injection is being performed so as to detect inadvertent vessel puncture

Never using adrenaline-containing solutions in areas supplied by end arteries e.g. fingers and toes, the penis

Local anaesthetic blocks should never be performed if resuscitation equipment is not immediately available.

Respiratory depression is treated with oxygen and artificial ventilation as appropriate.

Cardiovascular collapse is treated with oxygen, the rapid administration of intravenous fluids, a head-down tilt, vasoconstrictors (e.g. ephedrine, metaraminol) and atropine. In severe cases, external cardiac massage may be necessary.

Convulsions are treated with oxygen and intravenous diazepam.

Local Anaesthetic Agents

Only three local anaesthetic agents are in widespread use in the UK at present. They are presented both as plain solutions and with added adrenaline or, in the case of prilocaine, felypressin. The latter agents are added to the local anaesthetic solution to produce local vasoconstriction which will slow absorption thus prolonging the duration of the block and reducing the risk of toxic side-effects. Remember a 1% solution contains 10 mg/ml.

Lignocaine. The standard agent with which others tend to be compared. It is rapidly effective and lasts for 60-90 min. A 1% solution will produce a sensory block of most nerves. More concentrated solutions are available if motor blockade is also required, and for topical use on mucous membranes (e.g. the urethra and larynx). The maximum recommended adult dose is of the order of 200 mg of the plain solution and 400–500 mg of the adrenaline-containing solution.

Prilocaine. This is generally similar to lignocaine but with a greater therapeutic index. Larger amounts may, therefore, be used – 300 mg of the plain solution and up to 600 mg of the felypressin or adrenaline-containing solutions. Plain solutions of prilocaine are specifically indicated for intravenous regional anaesthesia (Bier's block).

Bupivacaine. The local anaesthetic with the longest duration of action, it is also the most potent and the most toxic. It is presented as 0.25%, 0.5% and 0.75% solutions. The maximum recommended dose is in the order of 2–3 mg/kg in any 4 h period.

Specific Local Anaesthetic Blocks

Spinal Blockade

Spinals are among the simplest yet most reliable local anaesthetic blocks to perform. The dura mater (theca) is punctured below the level at which the spinal cord usually ends (L2) and 2–3 ml of local anaesthetic solution injected. Spinals are generally reserved for operations on the lower half of the body, such as prostatic and hip surgery, because if large volumes of local anaesthetic are injected to obtain a more extensive block, excessive sympathetic blockade and profound hypotension can occur.

Hypotension due to sympathetically mediated vasodilatation is probably the commonest complication of spinal anaesthesia. A moderate degree of hypotension in a well-oxygenated, supine patient is of no great consequence and may well reduce operative blood loss. In a conscious patient, nausea often occurs if too great a degree of hypotension is allowed to develop. Profound hypotension will result in impaired tissue perfusion and should be treated vigorously with intravenous fluids and vasoconstrictors.

A further complication peculiar to spinal anaesthesia is headache. This is thought to occur because cerebrospinal fluid (c.s.f.) continues to leak through the hole in the dura produced by the original needle puncture. If the headache is severe and does not settle with bed rest, it is now common practice to perform an epidural blood patch; blood is aspirated aseptically from the patient and then injected into the epidural space, just outside the theca, where it forms a clot and seals the leak. The headache is generally quickly and dramatically relieved.

Epidural Blockade

Epidural blocks are now widely used to provide pain relief during labour and are becoming increasingly popular as the sole anaesthetic for operations such as caesarean section or hip replacement. They may also be used in conjunction with a general anaesthetic for lengthy and painful procedures, such as abdomino-perineal resections, both to lower blood pressure and reduce blood loss and to provide post-operative analgesia.

Catheters are frequently inserted into the epidural space so that either regular boluses or a continuous infusion of local anaesthetic can be given to provide post-operative analgesia. Two life-threatening complications can occur with this technique. If the catheter erodes the dura mater and passes intrathecally, a profound and extensive sensory and motor block will result. Hypotension, bradycardia and respiratory paralysis will follow. The treatment of this dramatic complication is simple. Vasoconstrictors and fluids are used to treat the hypotension, atropine is given for the bradycardia and oxygen and artificial ventilation administered until the patient is able to breathe again. The second major complication occurs if the catheter punctures a blood vessel and the local anaesthetic is given intravenously. Convulsions can occur and they are treated with intravenous diazepam and oxygen as outlined previously.

Other less dramatic problems, however, are more commonly encountered:

Some degree of motor blockade often occurs and the patient will have difficulty and need help in altering their position.

Patients may be unaware of the position of their anaesthetised limbs. Care must be taken to ensure that such limbs are carefully positioned and not inadvertently damaged.

Bladder sensation may be lost and retention of urine can result. Micturition can sometimes be initiated by pressure over the bladder but catheterisation may be necessary.

Patients should be warned not to attempt to get out of bed or they may collapse from a combination of hypotension and leg muscle weakness.

Epidural Narcotics

It has recently been shown that if narcotics rather than local anaesthetics are injected epidurally, analgesia without motor, sensory or sympathetic blockade can be obtained. This is believed to occur because the narcotics bind locally to receptors in the cord that normally respond to the body's own endorphins. The dose of narcotic required is similar to that given intravenously but its duration of action is often much greater; a single dose of, say, morphine might last for 12 hours or more. Generally, the quality of the analgesia produced is better than that produced by narcotics given by more conventional routes. Side-effects, however, are similar and respiratory depression is the most important and can occur insidiously many hours after the drug was given. The treatment of such respiratory depression is, however, exactly the same as that which follows conventional narcotics and naloxone should be given intravenously. Interestingly in such circumstances, naloxone reverses respiratory depression but not analgesia, presumably because it is not present in a high enough concentration to displace the narcotic from its cord receptors. A further curious but less dangerous side-effect is nasal itching. It, too, is controlled by naloxone.

Caudal Blockade

A caudal is essentially the same as an epidural in that local anaesthetic is injected into the epidural space. The only real difference is that caudal injections are given through the sacro-coccygeal membrane which overlies the epidural space where the bodies of the lower two sacral vertebrae (S4, S5) fail to fuse in the midline rather than between two lumbar vertebrae. Technically, they are easier to perform than lumbar epidurals but are only suitable for a limited range of perineal operations. They offer excellent peri-operative and post-operative analgesia for such procedures as circumcision, hernia repair, orchidopexy and haemorrhoidectomy.

Although inadvertent intrathecal or intravascular injection are theoretical complications, the problems most likely to be encountered post-operatively are urinary retention and muscle weakness in the legs. As caudals are frequently performed in children, patients should be reassured that nothing dreadful has happened to them if they experience these side-effects.

Local Infiltration

Increasingly surgeons are infiltrating the wound with a long-acting local anaesthetic (e.g. bupivacaine) before they suture the skin. This provides useful analgesia after many operations. Complications rarely occur but the patient may still need a narcotic as the local anaesthetic will only block discomfort from skin and muscle and not that due to trauma to bone or intra-abdominal structures.

Intercostal Nerve Blockade

Each intercostal nerve emerges through an intervertebral foramen and initially runs with an artery and vein behind the rib after which it is named. The upper six nerves innervate the chest wall, while the lower six supply the abdominal wall. Generally, the fourth nerve (T4) supplies skin at about the level of the nipple, the sixth nerve (T6) supplies the area at the level of the xiphisternum, the tenth (T10), the level of the umbilicus and the twelfth nerve (T12), that above the pubis.

Intercostal nerve blockade produces excellent analgesia for fractured ribs and can produce useful pain relief for most thoracic and upper abdominal incisions, particularly if they are unilateral. If an incision is in the midline, bilateral nerve blocks are needed and the amount of local anaesthetic required may approach toxic levels. In addition, bilateral blockade may produce intercostal and abdominal muscle weakness and make breathing difficult for those with chronic obstructive airways disease.

The principal complication of intercostal nerve blockade is pneumothorax but most pneumothoraces produced when attempting this block are small and need no treatment. However, if any patient becomes cyanosed or restless or has difficulty in breathing after intercostal nerve blockade, a significant pneumothorax should be suspected and a chest X-ray taken immediately. If the suspicion is confirmed, it may be necessary to insert a chest drain although this is a rare occurrence.

Intrapleural Catheterisation

Recently there has been some interest in inserting intrapleural catheters when prolonged analgesia is required or post-operative pain is likely to be severe. With this technique the pleura is deliberately punctured and a catheter inserted between the parietal and visceral pleura. Local anaesthetic can then be injected through the catheter at regular intervals or a continuous infusion given by a syringe pump. This technique would seem to be particularly valuable following thoracic surgery or when a patient has multiple fractured ribs.

Inguinal Field Blockade

Analgesia for inguinal hernia repair may be obtained by blocking the relevant nerves in the groin. This is done by injecting local anaesthetic fan-wise through the abdominal muscles medial to the iliac crest and again lateral to the pubic tubercle. It is wise to inject further local anaesthetic along the line of the proposed skin incision and again for the surgeon to inject more local anaesthetic around the neck of the hernial sac once it has been exposed.

Complications are few as long as excessive amounts of local anaesthetic are not used. If a long-acting agent such as bupivacaine is used, useful post-operative analgesia is obtained. This is a particularly valuable technique for day case surgery and for use on frail, elderly patients.

Penile Nerve Blockade

This is a block frequently performed in young boys undergoing circumcision or hypospadias repair. Local anaesthetic is injected around the dorsal nerves of the penis just below the pubic bone taking care not to inject into the vascular corpora cavernosa. Further local anaesthetic should be injected subcutaneously around the base of the penis.

If intravascular injection is avoided this block is usually without complication and provides excellent post-operative analgesia. It is imperative that adrenaline-containing solutions of local anaesthetic are not used for this block as any resulting arterial constriction would have devastating consequences!

Brachial Plexus Blockade

The brachial plexus is formed mainly from the roots of the 5th cervical to the 1st thoracic (C5–T1) nerves. It supplies sensation and motor power to the shoulder and arm. Although many methods of blocking the plexus have been described, two, the supraclavicular and the axillary, are in common use.

With the supraclavicular route, the plexus is blocked in the neck when it lies between the scalene muscles. Potentially, the whole plexus may be blocked and thus analgesia of the whole upper limb and shoulder obtained. With this method, there is a slight risk of pneumothorax. As the axillary name suggests, the plexus may also be blocked in the axilla when the nerves lie in close association with the axillary artery. There is then no risk of pneumothorax, but the upper roots which supply the shoulder will not be blocked.

A large variety of orthopaedic and soft tissue procedures can be carried out under brachial plexus block but it is especially indicated in patients with chronic renal failure who need an arteriovenous shunt to be fashioned prior to dialysis. Not only does such a block avoid the risks of general anaesthesia in these ill patients but the vasodilatation that follows sympathetic blockade makes the surgeon's task easier.

Occasionally, a continuous brachial plexus block may be performed after a catheter is inserted into the plexus sheath. The analgesia and vasodilatation produced is especially useful in those patients who have had reconstructive surgery involving microvascular anastamoses.

Patients who have had a brachial plexus block are often unaware of the position of their arm while it is anaesthetised. It is, therefore, important that during recovery the arm is always positioned in such a way that it cannot be inadvertently damaged.

Intravenous Regional Anaesthesia (Bier's Block)

At the turn of the century, Bier described an alternative method of anaesthetising the upper limb. If a tourniquet inflated to a pressure greater than systolic is inflated around the upper arm and local anaesthetic solution injected intravenously in the hand, that part of the limb distal to the tourniquet will be anaesthetised. Fractures may then be reduced and minor surgery performed on the anaesthetised limb.

This method of producing analgesia is much easier to perform than brachial plexus blockade and so has become very popular. It is, however, not without its hazards and several patients have died when the block has been performed by practitioners who were unaware of its complications or who were unable to treat them. Difficulties are likely to occur if the tourniquet leaks or deflates suddenly soon after the local anaesthetic has been injected. The end result is the same as if the local anaesthetic were injected directly intravenously and convulsions and cardiovascular depression will follow. The treatment is as outlined above. It is, therefore, imperative that the tourniquet be checked carefully before starting the block and that it is monitored throughout the procedure.

Two further problems may commonly occur:

The patient may complain of pain from the unanaesthetised area beneath the tourniquet if the procedure is prolonged. This can be best managed by using two tourniquets, one above the other. The more proximal tourniquet is first inflated and when it becomes painful, the distal tourniquet inflated on the analgesic area below it and the proximal cuff deflated.

When the tourniquet is deflated, some local anaesthetic will still be free in the veins. As it enters the systemic circulation, toxic effects may occur. These may include ringing in the ears, dizziness, a metallic taste in the mouth or nausea. The longer the tourniquet has been inflated, the less troublesome are these side-effects. Their incidence can also be reduced by slowing the release of the residual local anaesthetic into the circulation by re-inflating and deflating the tourniquet cuff a number of times.

This method of local anaesthesia can also be applied to the leg but larger volumes of local anaesthetic are required with a greater potential for toxic reactions.

Digital Nerve Blockade

Individual digits, be they fingers or toes, can be easily blocked by injecting small amounts of local anaesthetic into the web space on either side of the digit where the digital nerves run. Foreign bodies or ingrowing nails may then painlessly be removed or lacerations sutured.

As digits are supplied by end arteries, adrenaline-containing solutions should not be used or ischaemic gangrene may result.

Femoral Nerve Blockade

This is probably the most useful block that can be performed on the leg. The femoral nerve lies lateral to the femoral artery as they both pass beneath the inguinal ligament and enter the thigh. An isolated femoral nerve block produces an area of analgesia in the thigh but, more importantly, can relieve the pain of a fractured shaft of femur.

If a larger volume of local anaesthetic is injected it will track up in the same fascial plane as the femoral nerve and block the obturator and lateral cutaneous nerve of the thigh as well: a 3-in-1 block. Such a block is indicated when split skin grafts are taken from the antero-lateral aspect of the thigh. This donor site can be extremely painful and a 3-in-1 block can render it totally pain free.

Patient Management in the Recovery Unit

Many of the specific complications of local anaesthetic blocks have been mentioned above. Most occur at, or soon after, the local anaesthetic is injected and so are not likely to be seen in the recovery room.

A number of potentially major problems may be encountered by recovery unit staff.

1. If catheters have been inserted and top-ups are given in the recovery room, problems may be encountered even if the original injection was uneventful. Catheters are most commonly inserted in the epidural space but they may move intrathecally or intravascularly. A top-up may, therefore, respectively result in either a total spinal block with profound hypotension and muscle paralysis or convulsions. Although aspiration on the catheter before injection may reveal c.s.f. or blood, nothing may be aspirated before the injection is given.

It matters not one iota whether the injection is given by a consultant anaesthetist, a syringe pump or a well-trained chimpanzee. What is really important is who is with the patient after the injection and whether they can recognise and treat the complications that may occur. An observant and well-trained nurse is essential for the well-being of the patient.

2. Patients who have had major blocks (epidurals and spinals) may have a significant residual sympathetic block after the motor and sensory block has disappeared. This may result in hypotension and fainting if such patients try to sit or stand soon after the block. All changes of position should take place gradually and the blood pressure should be checked frequently.

3. Those areas of the patient's body that remain affected by a sensory block should be protected against inadvertent injury. Arms and legs are particularly vulnerable and must always be positioned appropriately. Both the patient and the ward staff need to be reminded to exercise due care.

It is self evident that when the patient is transferred to the care of the ward staff, they are told that a local block has been performed and the degree to which the patient is still affected by it. They may need to be reminded of potential problems that may occur if local anaesthetic blocks are infrequently performed on patients in their care.

Further Reading

Alexander JI, Hill RG (1987) Postoperative pain control. Blackwell Scientific Publications, London
Cousins MJ, Bridenbaugh PO (1980) Neural blockade in clinical anaesthesia and management of pain. Lippincott, Philadelphia
Cousins MJ, Philips GD (1986) Acute pain management. Churchill Livingstone, London
Eriksson E (1969) Illustrated handbook in local anaesthesia. Munksgaard, Copenhagen
Wildsmith JAW, Armitage EN (1987) Principles and practice of regional anaesthesia. Churchill Livingstone, London

Chapter 4
Complications

Respiratory Complications

The function of the respiratory system is the delivery of oxygen to, and the elimination of carbon dioxide from the blood. Any respiratory complication will, if uncorrected, lead to inadequate oxygenation (hypoxaemia) and/or retention of CO_2 (hypercarbia), and these conditions must be readily recognised by recovery staff. The incidence of such problems is greater after lengthy anaesthesia and surgery.

Signs of hypoxaemia

1. Cyanosis. This may be difficult to detect in the presence of anaemia or poor peripheral perfusion
2. Restlessness and confusion. This indicates impaired cerebral oxygenation
3. Tachycardia followed by bradycardia

Signs of hypercarbia

1. Tachycardia
2. Hypertension
3. Sweating
4. Irregular pulse, especially pulsus bigeminus
5. Flushed skin due to capillary vasodilatation. (This may give a mistaken impression of well-being)
6. Clouding of consciousness

The increased use of pulse oximeters allows hypoxaemia to be recognised early before cyanosis develops. The diagnosis may be confirmed by taking a sample of arterial blood for blood gas analysis.

Upper Airway Obstruction

Partial obstruction of the airway may be indicated by:

1. Stertorous breathing i.e. snoring
2. Inspiratory stridor i.e. a crowing noise on inspiration
3. Laboured breathing. Use of the accessory muscles of respiration (sterno-mastoids, scalenes) with retraction of the head on inspiration and flaring of the nostrils
4. Rocking movements of the abdomen and chest. Instead of the abdomen and chest rising and falling in phase together, downward descent of the diaphragm with abdominal distension is accompanied by retraction or indrawing of the thorax, creating a see-saw or rocking motion of the chest and abdomen (external paradoxical respiration). This becomes more marked as the degree of obstruction increases

If respiratory obstruction is complete:

1. No movement of air is detectable at the airway
2. There are no breath sounds
3. Signs of hypoxia rapidly develop
4. Dysrhythmias and bradycardia occur

It is important to note that movements of the chest are not synonymous with a clear airway; indeed, excessive chest movements may occur in the presence of complete airway obstruction. Remember also that although partial obstruction is accompanied by noisy respiration, total obstruction is silent.

Causes

1. *Tongue.* In the unconscious patient with the jaw relaxed the tongue may fall back and obstruct the airway.
2. *Foreign material in the pharynx*
   a) Excess mucous or saliva
   b) Gastric contents from vomiting or regurgitation
   c) Blood following oral or nasal surgery
   d) Broken or dislodged teeth
   e) Dental packs not removed before extubation.
3. *Laryngospasm.* Resulting from stimulation of the larynx during emergence from anaesthesia. This may be caused by foreign material (as above) or by clumsy extubation or suction.

The following are less common but nevertheless potentially lethal:

4. *Laryngeal oedema* following trauma, intubation or infection. This is especially dangerous in the young, when the airway is of narrow diameter.

5. *External pressure on the trachea.*
   a) Haematoma following thyroid surgery or following attempts at internal jugular cannulation
   b) Use of constrictive Elastoplast bandages.
6. *Abductor paralysis of vocal cords.* This may occur following damage to the recurrent laryngeal nerve during thyroid surgery (see p. 121).
7. *Tracheal collapse* following thyroidectomy.

Management

1. Extend the neck
2. Lift the jaw forward
3. Insert an oral airway. If the teeth are tightly clenched due to spasm of the masseters, firm pressure on the mandible may be necessary to enable the airway to be inserted. If this fails a nasopharyngeal airway may be inserted to bypass the obstruction. If the obstruction remains unrelieved, foreign material in the pharynx must be suspected. If the patient is not already on his side then:
4. Turn the patient on to his side (preferably his left in case subsequent laryngoscopy becomes necessary)
5. Tilt head down (Trendelenburg position) to help clear any foreign material
6. Apply suction to pharynx with rigid Yankauer sucker or large suction catheter

If these measures are unsuccessful proceed to:

7. Laryngoscopy – so that foreign material can be sucked out under direct vision or removed using Magill forceps. If the larynx is clear but the vocal cords are in spasm:
8. Give oxygen by anaesthetic face mask and Mapleson C circuit (Fig. 2.14). Apply gentle pressure to the reservoir bag to try and overcome the spasm. If this is unsuccessful, give intravenous suxamethonium (succinylcholine) to relax the cords and ventilate the lungs. Endotracheal intubation may be necessary.

Special consideration will be required for the less common causes of stridor (nos. 4–7 above):

Laryngeal oedema. Although this usually resolves spontaneously, preparations for rapid intubation should be made. The following may aid spontaneous resolution:

a) Head up position to improve venous drainage
b) Humidification
c) Steroids
d) Diuretics
e) Inhalation of nebulised adrenaline (racemic epinephrine)

The inhalation of a mixture of helium 80% and oxygen 20% will reduce the resistance to air flow and make breathing easier.

External pressure on the trachea ⎫
Abductor paralysis of vocal cords ⎬ See complications of thyroid
Tracheal collapse   ⎭ surgery (p. 121)

Inadequate Ventilation (Hypoventilation)

If correction of upper airway obstruction does not lead to the resumption of a normal breathing pattern or if signs of hypoxaemia or hypercarbia develop, then inadequate alveolar ventilation must be suspected. If there is doubt, confirmation can be obtained by:

1. *Attaching a pulse oximeter* to the patient's finger or ear lobe. Usually, the haemoglobin saturation is greater than 95%.
2. *Measuring the respiratory minute volume,* using a Wright's spirometer (normal values should exceed 5 litres/minute). Because of the difficulty of obtaining an airtight fit with a mask, this method may be unsatisfactory in patients who are not intubated.
3. *Analysing blood gases* on an arterial sample. Inadequate alveolar ventilation is characterised by a respiratory acidosis (pH < 7.35, $PaCO_2$ > 6kPa).

Except in an emergency, when intubation and controlled ventilation must be instituted without delay, an attempt should be made to determine the cause of the inadequate ventilation so that specific treatment aimed at correcting this may be undertaken.

Causes

Causes of inadequate ventilation in the immediate post-operative period are:

1. Depression of the respiratory centre/Cheyne-Stokes respiration
2. Residual muscle paralysis
3. Interference with the mechanics of respiration

Depression of Respiratory Centre

Depression of the respiratory centre may be due to:

1. Drugs
   a) Opiates given before or during anaesthesia
   b) Barbiturates
   c) Inhalation agents

2. Lack of respiratory drive
   a) Low $PaCO_2$ following hyperventilation during anaesthesia
   b) Loss of hypoxic drive due to administrations of high concentrations of oxygen to patients suffering from chronic pulmonary disease

Central depression may be suspected by:

1. Delayed return of consciousness. Patients should normally show signs of returning consciousness within 15 min of arrival in the recovery room
2. Respiratory rate below 10 breaths/minute with a low tidal volume
3. Constricted pupils following opiate administration
4. History of chronic pulmonary disease

Management. If central depression due to opiates is suspected, this may be corrected by either of the following:

1. Intravenous naloxone, 0.1–0.4 mg. This drug is a specific opiate antagonist and is therefore ineffective in other forms of respiratory depression. It should be given slowly in increments of 0.1 mg every 2–3 min and its effect titrated against the patient's respiratory response. Excessive doses will reverse not only the respiratory depression but also the analgesic effect of the opiates, causing the patient unnecessary pain. To extend the duration of action, subsequent injections can be given by the intramuscular route.
2. Intravenous doxapram, 1 mg/kg. This drug is a direct stimulant of the respiratory centre and has advantages over naloxone as it is effective for other causes of central respiratory depression and does not reverse analgesia.

Since the depressant effects of the opiates may outlast either of these antidotes, they may have to be repeated.

If there is a history of pulmonary disease, graded concentrations of oxygen should be given using a Venturi mask and progress monitored by repeated blood gas analysis.

If the situation does not improve, it is safer to intubate the trachea and electively ventilate the lungs until the effects of anaesthesia and surgery have worn off.

Cheyne-Stokes Respiration

This is an irregular pattern of respiration characterised by periods of hyperventilation alternating with hypoventilation. It is more commonly seen in elderly patients. Causes of Cheyne-Stokes respiration are:

1. Left ventricular failure
2. Depression of respiratory centre
3. Raised intracranial pressure
4. Uraemia

Management. This condition may be aggravated by the administration of sedative drugs which should be used with caution in the recovery period.

An underlying condition should be sought and treated if possible. If respiration becomes inadequate, intubation and controlled ventilation will be required.

Residual Paralysis

Residual paralysis may be due to the continued action of muscle relaxants given during anaesthesia causing neuromuscular block of either the depolarising or non-depolarising type. Residual paralysis should be suspected if there is:

1. Laboured breathing – use of accessory muscles of respiration (extension of neck on inspiration)
2. Rapid shallow breathing with minimal chest movement
3. Flaring of the nostrils and/or raising of the eyebrows
4. Unexplained restlessness
5. The patient whispers that he cannot breathe properly
6. Tracheal tug (downward movement of trachea and thyroid cartilage on inspiration)

Simple bedside tests to indicate residual paralysis

1. Ask the patient to grip your hand, raise his head from the pillow or protrude his tongue for several seconds.
2. Measure his vital capacity: normal value should exceed 10 ml/kg

The type of treatment will depend on whether the residual paralysis is due to a depolarising (phase I) or non-depolarising (phase II) block. A knowledge of the type, quantity and timing of the muscle relaxants given during anaesthesia will usually clarify this but if doubt remains additional information may be obtained from:

1. *Peripheral nerve stimulation.* If a train of four supramaximal stimuli at a frequency of 2 Hz is applied to the ulnar nerve, contraction of the hand muscles will result. This is painful for the conscious patient and should not be applied more frequently than is essential. Fade with successive stimuli confirms non-depolarising block (Fig. 4. 1). Significant paralysis is indicated if the ratio of the fourth to the first response is less than 50%.
2. *Edrophonium test.* An intravenous injection of the short-acting anticholinesterase drug edrophonium will increase muscle strength if the patient has a non-depolarising block. It is unwise to use the longer-acting neostigmine as it will exacerbate a depolarising block.

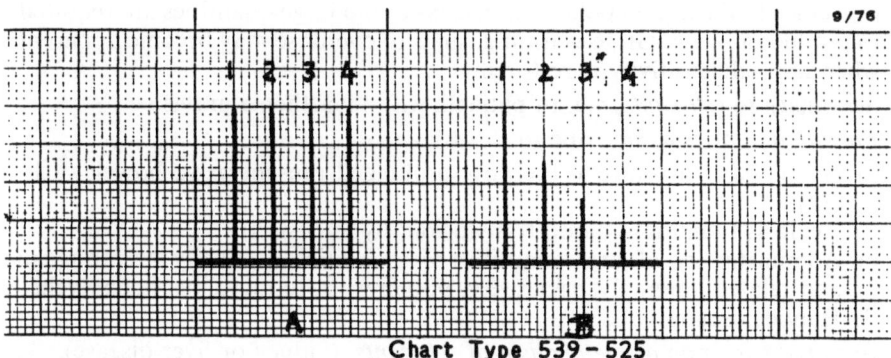

Fig. 4.1. Results of train of four stimulation. A, normal response; B, fade of successive stimuli

Depolarising Block (Phase I Block)

Suxamethonium (succinylcholine) is normally metabolised by cholinesterase in the blood within 5–10 min of administration with the resumption of spontaneous respiration. Paralysis is prolonged in the presence of:

1. *Abnormal cholinesterase.* A rare inherited condition in which there is an impaired ability to metabolise suxamethonium
2. *Reduced amounts of cholinesterase.* Cholinesterase is synthesised in the liver and may be deficient in liver disease or malnutrition
3. *Concurrent administration of anticholinesterases,* e.g. ecothiopate (phospholine iodide) used in the treatment of glaucoma

Management of Phase I Block. If, following the administration of suxamethonium (succinylcholine), spontaneous respiration has not returned by the time the patient arrives in the recovery unit, assisted ventilation must be continued. Spontaneous respiration is normally resumed within 2 hours but can be expedited by the administration of cholinesterase in the form of fresh frozen plasma.

Before the patient leaves hospital, blood should be taken for estimation of cholinesterase level and dibucaine number. If abnormal cholinesterase is demonstrated by a low dibucaine number (normal 80%), the family practitioner must be notified and other members of the family investigated as they may also be affected.

Non-depolarising Block (Phase II Block)

Non-depolarising block may be due to:

1. *Excessive administration of non-depolarising relaxants* in relation to the patient's size and the duration of surgery. During hypothermia there is

resistance to the non-depolarising relaxants and large quantities are required to produce a block. On re-warming, signs of overdose may become apparent when normal sensitivity is restored.

2. *Sensitivity to relaxants,* e.g. in patients with myasthenia gravis
3. *Potentiation of relaxants* due to:
   a) Hypokalaemia (diuretic therapy, prolonged pre-operative bowel wash-out)
   b) Acidosis (vomiting, blood transfusion, hypotension)
   c) Administration of large quantities of antibiotics, especially streptomycin and related aminoglycosides, e.g. polymyxins, tetracycline, lincomycin
   d) Hypocalcaemia
4. *Impaired excretion or metabolism of relaxants* (kidney or liver disease)
5. *Excessive administration of depolarising relaxants.* When the amount of suxamethonium (succinylcholine) administered exceeds 300 mg the depolarising block (phase I) may develop into a non-depolarising (phase II) block

Management of Phase II Block

1. Administer intravenous neostigmine (preceded by atropine or glycopyrolate) to a total dose, including that given at the end of surgery, of 0.08 mg/kg. If this does not reverse the neuromuscular block, controlled ventilation is continued while further attempts are made to determine the cause.
2. Take blood for blood gas and electrolyte estimation.
3. Correct metabolic acidosis with intravenous sodium bicarbonate using the formula: base deficit × body weight in kg × 1/3 = mmol of sodium bicarbonate required. This is normally given in several increments and the effect measured by serial blood gas estimations.
4. Correct hypokalaemia by intravenous potassium chloride. Up to 20 mmol of a dilute solution may be given per hour with continuous ECG monitoring.
5. If hypocalcaemia is suspected following massive transfusion of stored blood, or if large quantities of antibiotics have been given, 10 ml of 10% calcium chloride intravenously may correct the situation.

Conditions Affecting the Mechanics of Respiration

Inadequate ventilation may occur post-operatively if respiratory movements are impaired by:

1. Pain from a high abdominal or thoracic incision
2. Obesity (p. 158)
3. Tight abdominal or thoracic strapping
4. Pneumothorax or haemothorax

Management

1. Give oxygen by face mask to increase the inspired oxygen concentration (F_1O_2)
2. Sit patient up to lessen pressure on diaphragm
3. Ensure adequate analgesia
4. Encourage deep breathing by means of physiotherapy

If the history or clinical findings suggest pneumothorax or haemothorax, an X-ray of the chest should be taken and appropriate management instituted (p. 78).

Progress can be monitored by serial blood gas estimation. If there is no improvement with the above measures, intubation and controlled ventilation will be required.

Hypoxaemia

Causes

In addition to the hypoxaemia resulting from generalised underventilation of the lungs and a reduced respiratory minute volume (p. 70), it may also be caused post-operatively by the following:

1. *Diffusion hypoxaemia* (Fink effect). In the first few minutes after nitrous oxide is discontinued, it comes out of solution in the blood and diffuses into the alveoli. The concentration of oxygen is, therefore, reduced below normal if the patient is breathing room air. Oxygen should always be administered after nitrous oxide is discontinued.
2. *Increased oxygen utilisation* accompanying shivering, convulsions, pyrexia, thyroid crisis
3. *Ventilation perfusion (V:Q) imbalance* caused by regional underventilation. Some alveoli continue to receive a normal blood supply but are not adequately ventilated. This occurs if there is atelectasis due to:
   a) Absorption collapse distal to an obstruction caused by plugs of mucus or inhalation of foreign material
   b) Surgical compression of the lung during thoracotomy
   c) Airway closure at the bases due to pain causing restricted movements
   d) Pneumonia
   e) Pulmonary oedema

Management

1. Administer oxygen by face mask to increase the proportion of inspired oxygen (F_1O_2). This is particularly important in the elderly and in those with a reduced cardiopulmonary reserve

If atelectasis is the likely cause:

2. Encourage deep breathing and arrange regular physiotherapy
3. Ensure there is adequate analgesia
4. Monitor progress by serial blood gas estimations

Bronchospasm

In spontaneously breathing patients, bronchospasm is characterised by dyspnoea and wheezing, especially during expiration. In patients being ventilated, an increased airway pressure is required to inflate the lungs (decreased compliance).

Causes

1. *Predominance of parasympathetic tone*, e.g. following neostigmine or non-selective β-blockers such as propranolol
2. *Irritation of larynx* during emergence from anaesthesia, e.g. by secretions, gastric contents, endotracheal tube, suction catheter. Chronic bronchitics and smokers are especially prone to this problem
3. *Anaphylactoid reactions* due to histamine release following administration of drugs such as *d*-tubocurarine and Haemaccel or following blood transfusion
4. *Asthma*

Management

1. Administration of oxygen
2. Bronchodilators, e.g. aminophylline 250–500 mg intravenously given slowly to minimise tachycardia *or* salbutamol (albuterol) either intravenously or via nebuliser (see Fig. 4.2)
3. Hydrocortisone 100 mg i.v. to reduce mucosal swelling

If bronchospasm and dyspnoea persist despite these measures:

4. Intubate and ventilate the lungs

Aspiration of Gastric Contents

During recovery from general anaesthesia the laryngeal reflex may be depressed. Therefore, if vomiting or regurgitation occurs, gastric contents may be aspirated into the trachea and lungs. To reduce this risk patients recovering from

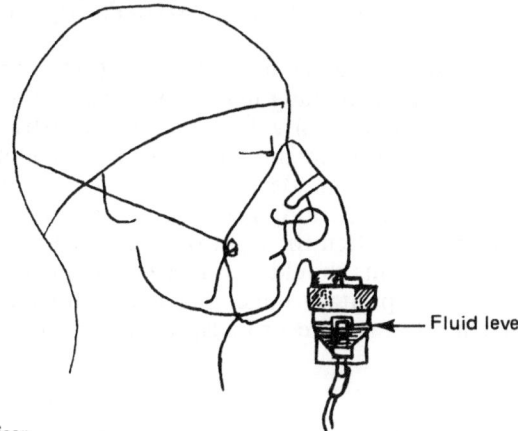

Fig. 4.2. Drug administration via nebuliser.

anaesthesia are normally nursed on the side so that regurgitated gastric contents do not pool in the posterior pharynx but are cleared with the aid of gravity.

If vomiting occurs during the recovery period:

1. *Turn patient on to side* if not already in this position. The left side is preferable since if the patient is supine, inhaled material may normally enter the right lung and drainage will be facilitated with this lung uppermost. Also subsequent laryngoscopy is easiest with the patient on the left side
2. *Tilt bed head down* (Trendelenburg position)
3. *Apply suction to pharynx.* Laryngoscopy and Magill forceps may be required to remove solid material
4. *Give oxygen by face mask*

If aspiration has occurred:

5. *Intubate* and give 100% oxygen
6. *Apply suction* to the trachea and main bronchi using a fine catheter via the endotracheal tube
7. *Consider bronchoscopy* if hypoxia persists or if solid material has been inhaled
8. *Give bronchodilators* as required to relieve bronchospasm (see p. 76)
9. *Administer hydrocortisone* 100–500 mg i.v. to reduce mucosal swelling
10. *Encourage coughing* and arrange vigorous physiotherapy in an attempt to clear the lungs

Antibiotics are not usually recommended at this stage, as gastric contents are usually sterile, but may be added if pyrexia develops or when the results of sputum culture become known. An early X-ray of the chest may provide a baseline for subsequent comparison.

Chemical Pneumonitis (Mendelson's Syndrome)

If the gastric contents are highly acid (pH < 2.5), as may occur during labour, aspiration into the lung may also cause chemical pneumonitis.

Aspiration of small volumes of acidic gastric contents may be silent and the signs of chemical pneumonitis may not develop for several hours. It must be suspected if a patient develops tachypnoea, cyanosis, tachycardia and wheezing in the recovery period. The chest X-ray may show diffuse opacities over the affected area, often the right base, thus confirming the diagnosis.

These patients should be transferred to an intensive care unit for management as severe respiratory difficulties may subsequently occur. The recovery room nurse must always record suspected regurgitation and vomiting.

Pneumothorax and Haemothorax

Pneumothorax (the presence of air in the pleural cavity) may become evident during recovery from anaesthesia. It is suggested by:

1. Chest pain
2. Dyspnoea
3. Cyanosis
4. Diminished air entry on affected side
5. Pulsus alternans

A chest X-ray will confirm the diagnosis.

Causes

1. Damage to pleura following surgery or trauma
2. Accidental pleural puncture following intercostal or supraclavicular brachial plexus block or during attempts at internal jugular or subclavian vein cannulation
3. Alveolar rupture during intermittent positive pressure ventilation or the spontaneous rupture of an emphysematous bulla

Management

A small pneumothorax unaccompanied by clinical features may resolve spontaneously and not require treatment.

A larger pneumothorax requires the insertion of a chest drain with underwater seal. A suitable site is the second interspace in the mid-clavicular line.

N.B. The administration of nitrous oxide in the presence of a pneumothorax will increase its size and should be avoided.

If the chest X-ray demonstrates the presence of fluid in the pleural cavity (haemothorax, pleural effusion), this should be released by a chest drain placed in the eighth space in the posterior axillary line.

Tension Pneumothorax

If the pneumothorax is under tension, the signs will be more acute. In addition there will be:

1. Cardiovascular collapse due to diminished venous return
2. Deviation of the trachea and displacement of the apex beat away from the affected side
3. Increasing difficulty in inflating the lungs in the ventilated patient

Management

Urgent insertion of a chest drain (see p. 128). In an emergency, the increased intrapleural pressure can be reduced rapidly by inserting a large-bore intravenous cannula into the second intercostal space while equipment is prepared for a more formal procedure.

Cardiovascular Complications

Hypotension

The post-operative blood pressure should not be considered in isolation but as part of a trend and interpreted in relation to the pulse rate and to other findings such as the pre-operative value and the state of the peripheral perfusion. For example, a reduction of 30 mmHg in the systolic pressure of a hypersensitive patient may be a significant fall yet still be within the normal range. On the other hand, in the presence of good peripheral perfusion, a blood pressure below the normal range may be satisfactory following certain anaesthetic techniques (p. 143).

A reduced blood pressure is frequently due to the continuing action of drugs used during anaesthesia (Table 4.1) and will usually revert to normal as the agents are eliminated. While patients are recovering from the effects of these agents, vasomotor tone may be impaired and with it the patient's ability to compensate for sudden changes in posture. A temporary fall in blood pressure may follow transfer of the patient from the operating table or the lowering of

Table 4.1 Drugs used during anaesthesia causing hypotension

1. *Myocardial depression*
   Inhalational anaesthetic agents, e.g. halothane, enflurane
   β-blocking agents, e.g. propranolol, labetolol
   Intravenous induction agents, e.g. thiopentone, propofol

2. *Diminished peripheral vascular resistance*
   Inhalational anaesthetic agents, e.g. isoflurane
   Sympathetic blockade:
   a) Ganglion-blocking agents, e.g. trimetaphan
   b) Local anaesthetic agents used for spinal or epidural anaesthesia

3. *Vasodilating drugs*: nitroglycerine, nitroprusside, chlorpromazine, droperidol, opiates

the legs from the lithotomy position and patients should not sit up until the effects of these agents have worn off.

If, on admission to the recovery unit, the systolic blood pressure is below 100 mmHg systolic, the patient's progress should be monitored carefully until normal values are restored. If peripheral perfusion is impaired, hypovolaemia and diminished cardiac output must be excluded.

Hypovolaemia

Hypotension and poor peripheral perfusion are accompanied by increasing heart rate, pallor, collapsed veins (a low central venous pressure reading will confirm this) and oliguria (urine output $< 0.5\,ml/(kg \cdot h)$).

Causes

1. Inadequate fluid replacement following pre-operative dehydration or prolonged surgery with bowel exposure
2. Inadequate replacement of blood

Management

1. Give oxygen by face mask to increase the percentage of oxygen inspired (F_1O_2)
2. Elevate foot of bed
3. Increase rate of intravenous infusion

N.B. Vasoconstricting agents are not recommended in the presence of hypovolaemia since they will further decrease tissue perfusion.

If there has been haemorrhage, a blood transfusion may be necessary. Until cross-matched blood is ready, the following substitutes may be used:

1. Haemaccel (a modified gelatin)
2. Hespan (a modified starch)
3. Human plasma protein fraction (HPPF)
4. Dextran 70. If cross-matching has not already been undertaken, a sample of blood should be taken first as dextran may interfere with subsequent cross-matching techniques

If hypotension, pallor and collapsed veins persist despite these measures then continued bleeding must be suspected. This may be either:

1. *Revealed*, e.g. blood in drainage bottles, bladder irrigation or on dressings and packs
2. *Concealed*, e.g. intra-abdominal

In either case the transfusion must be continued and the surgeon and anaesthetist notified as further surgery may be required. Alternatively, persistent bleeding may be due to a failure of coagulation and this may be suspected if a sample of blood in a plain tube does not clot within 10 min (see p. 104). Blood should then be taken for a formal coagulation screen.

Diminished Cardiac Output

If hypotension and poor peripheral perfusion are not due to hypovolaemia then a diminished cardiac output must be considered. This may be indicated by distended veins, a raised CVP and a falling pulse pressure. The last is the difference between the systolic and diastolic pressure and is normally about 40 mmHg.

Causes and Management

1. *Cardiac failure.* A review of the patient's previous medical history and the intra-operative fluid balance may suggest this possibility. Breathlessness, tachycardia and pulmonary and peripheral oedema may confirm it. Management will include:

   a) Oxygen therapy
   b) Posture (reverse Trendelenburg position)
   c) Diuretics
   d) Fluid restriction
   e) Inotropic support (dopamine, dobutamine, digoxin)
   f) Intubation and intermittent positive pressure ventilation (in extreme cases only)

2. *Myocardial infarction.* There may be a history of myocardial ischaemia or the classical description of chest pain may be present. However, infarction

can occur silently in patients with no previous history of cardiac disease. A 12-lead ECG should be performed and blood taken for enzyme studies. Although these may not contribute to the immediate management of the patient, they may provide a valuable baseline for future reference.

3. *Pulmonary embolus.* Although this is uncommon in the immediate post-operative period, pleuritic chest pain and haemoptysis may suggest this diagnosis. A chest X-ray and full ECG should be obtained. Treatment includes oxygen therapy, pain relief and heparinisation.

4. *Cardiac tamponade.* This may follow surgery or trauma in the region of the mediastinum or, rarely, perforation of the myocardium by a central venous or pulmonary artery catheter. Faint heart sounds and a rising CVP accompanied by a falling blood pressure may suggest this possibility. Widening of the mediastinum on chest X-ray will provide confirmation. Emergency treatment is by needle aspiration from below the xiphisternum but a formal thoracotomy may be necessary.

5. *Tension pneumothorax* (see p. 79).

Other Causes of Hypotension

If hypovolaemia and diminished cardiac output have been excluded and the cause of hypotension remains obscure, the following should be considered:

1. *Septicaemia.* Especially following bowel or urological surgery. This may be suspected by pyrexia, tachycardia, flushing, sweating or delirium. Management includes vigorous intravenous therapy to achieve and maintain normal venous pressure, and antibiotic and steroid therapy.

2. *Inadequate steroid cover.* For patients on long-term steroid therapy or with undiagnosed Addison's disease. Initial management will consist of fluid replacement and steroid therapy (p. 145).

3. *Mismatched blood transfusion.* Hypotension may accompany other signs of mismatched transfusion, such as pyrexia, urticaria, flushing, shivering, haematuria and persistent bleeding. The transfusion should be stopped immediately and samples of the transfused blood and patient's blood sent to the laboratory for further investigations (see p. 102).

4. *Pain.* Usually causes hypertension but hypotension is sometimes seen and may respond to the administration of analgesics.

Hypertension

Like pre-operative hypertension, this is not uncommon in the immediate post-operative period.

Causes

1. Pain
2. Distension of bladder
3. Respiratory depression with hypercarbia
4. Overtransfusion
5. Cardiovascular surgery
6. Drugs used during anaesthesia, e.g. ketamine, methoxamine, ephedrine
7. Underlying condition, e.g. phaeochromocytoma, hyperthyroidism, raised intracranial pressure, pre-eclamptic toxaemia

Management

Once pain, bladder distension and respiratory complications have been treated, the hypertension usually reverts to normal within 2 hours without the need for specific treatment. However, in those with coronary artery or cerebrovascular disease, excessive hypertension may cause myocardial ischaemia or cerebral haemorrhage and active management is required. Similarly, following vascular surgery hypertension will cause an unnecessary strain on the graft and should be avoided.

Numerous drugs are available to reduce blood pressure, for example:

1. Alpha-blocking agents, e.g. phentolamine, chlorpromazine
2. Ganglion-blocking agents, e.g. trimetaphan
3. Drugs acting directly on peripheral vessels, e.g. sodium nitroprusside nitroglycerine, hydralazine

In the presence of an accompanying tachycardia a combined α- and β- blocking agent such as labetalol may be useful.

It is important to exclude any of the underlying conditions which will require specific treatment, although in 30% of the patients no obvious cause can be found.

Bradycardia

Sinus Bradycardia

A heart rate of less than 60 per minute is normal in fit athletes but may signify an underlying condition requiring correction.

Causes

1. Continuing action of drugs used before or during anaesthesia, e.g. opiates, neostigmine, β-blocking agents (even when used as eye-drops), digoxin

2. High sympathetic blockade following spinal or epidural anaesthesia
3. Parasympathetic stimulation due to pain or pharyngeal suction.
4. Hypoxia
5. Raised intracranial pressure
6. Decreased metabolic rate due to hypothermia, hypothyroidism
7. Acute gastric dilatation.

Management

Intravenous atropine (0.5–2 mg) will usually correct any excessive parasympathetic tone or, alternatively, ephedrine may be used if there is an accompanying sympathetic blockade with hypotension.

If there is no response and hypoxia and raised intracranial pressure can be excluded, an ECG is required to differentiate between sinus bradycardia and heart block. In sinus bradycardia the PR interval is normal, i.e. less than 0.2 s (Fig. 4.3).

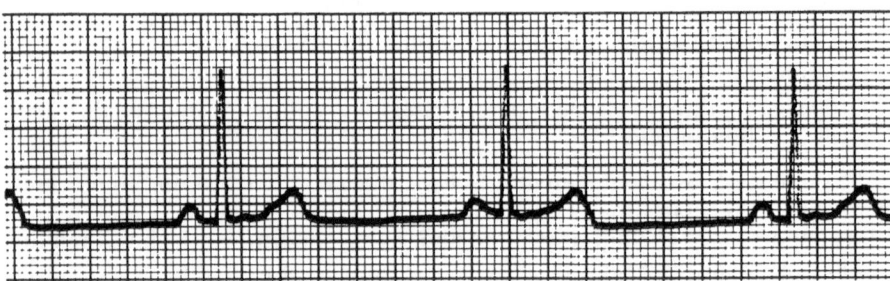

Fig. 4.3. Sinus bradycardia

Heart Block

Three types of heart block are identified on ECG.

1st degree heart block: PR interval greater than 0.2 s

2nd degree heart block: Mobitz type I (Wenckebach phenomenon). Gradual lengthening of PR interval until a dropped beat occurs. Mobitz type II. There is a failure of conduction so that only every 2nd or 3rd atrial impulse is conducted to the ventricles (2:1 or 3:1 block)

3rd degree heart block: Complete AV dissociation. No atrial impulses are conducted to the ventricles, which beat independently at a slow rate (Fig. 4.4)

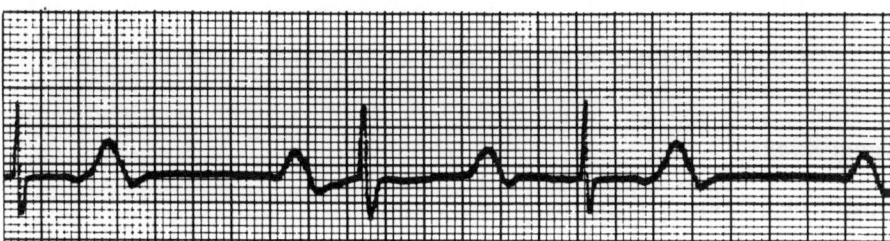

Fig. 4.4. Third degree heart block

Causes

1. Myocardial infarction
2. Drugs depressing myocardial conduction, e.g. digitalis, disopyramide, β-blocking agents

Management

Symptoms due to heart block, e.g. dizziness, fainting and poor peripheral perfusion, can frequently be treated by the infusion of a dilute solution of isoprenaline (isoproterenol) 4 mg in 500 ml 5% dextrose given via a paediatric infusion set. If this fails a pacemaker must be inserted.

Tachycardia

Sinus Tachycardia

There is a normal sinus rhythm but with a rate of over 100 per min.

A tachycardia is normal in infants and small children. Rates of up to 150 per min are well tolerated in patients with normal cardiac function and seldom require treatment but problems may arise in those with underlying heart disease because of the increased myocardial oxygen consumption and diminished stroke volume.

Causes

1. Pain
2. Respiratory problems causing hypercarbia or hypoxia
3. Circulatory disturbance, e.g. hypovolaemia, hypervolaemia
4. Infection
5. Drugs, e.g. atropine, ephedrine, adrenaline (epinephrine), ketamine

6. Anxiety
7. Underlying condition, e.g. hyperthyroidism, phaeochromocytoma

Management

Consists of treatment of the underlying cause.

1. Administer analgesics as required to relieve pain
2. Assess respiratory function using blood gas analysis if necessary. For treatment of inadequate ventilation, see p. 70
3. Assess circulation for signs of hypovolaemia or hypervolaemia:
   a) Hypovolaemia: cold clammy skin, thready pulse, collapsed veins, hypotension. Treat by fluid replacement
   b) Hypervolaemia: strong pulse, distended veins, normal or high blood pressure. Treat by fluid restriction, diuretics.
4. Give reassurance and add anxiolytics as required

Supraventricular and Ventricular Tachycardia (SVT and VT)

A heart rate in the region of 150–250 per min suggests either supraventricular or ventricular tachycardia. These may be accompanied by dizziness, palpitations, angina or chest pain and, if untreated, may lead to circulatory failure.

Causes

1. Hypoxia
2. Hypercarbia
3. Electrolyte disturbance, especially hypokalaemia
4. Acidosis
5. Coronary artery disease
6. Thyrotoxicosis

Management

1. Correct underlying cause if possible
2. Connect ECG monitor in order to distinguish supraventricular from ventricular tachycardia

Supraventricular tachycardia is characterised by normal QRS complexes. P waves may be abnormal or obscured by the T wave of the preceding complex (Fig. 4.5). Its management consists of:

1. Increasing vagal tone by carotid sinus massage, Valsalva manoeuvre or pressure on the eyeball

2. Verapamil 5-10 mg i.v.
3. Cardioversion using a synchronised DC shock. Further anaesthesia is necessary if consciousness has returned

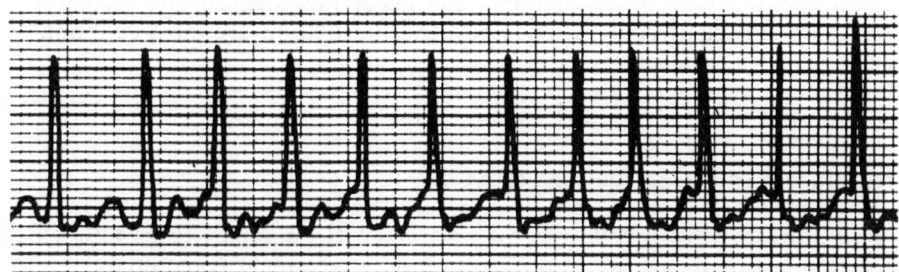

Fig. 4.5. Supraventricular tachycardia

Ventricular tachycardia is characterised by wide and abnormal QRS complexes and absence of P waves (Fig. 4.6). Treatment as listed below should be instituted without delay as ventricular fibrillation may follow.

1. Intravenous lignocaine (lidocaine) 1 mg/kg. If a ventricular tachycardia returns or there are frequent ventricular ectopic beats, a lignocaine infusion may be needed.
2. Flecainide 2 mg/kg over 20 min.
3. Cardioversion

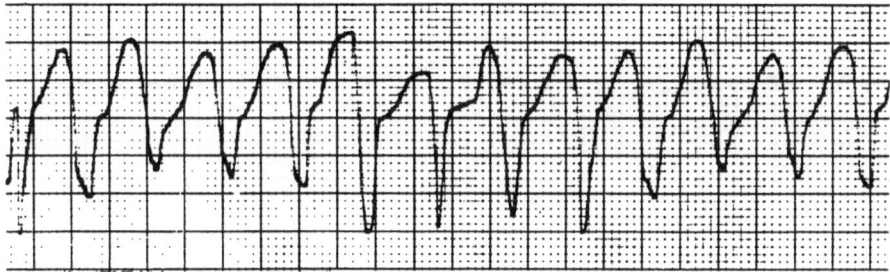

Fig. 4.6. Ventricular tachycardia

Dysrhythmias

An irregular pulse in the immediate post-operative period is not an uncommon finding, especially in children.

If the colour is good with the peripheral circulation satisfactory and the blood pressure maintained, no immediate treatment is required. The irregularity is probably due to residual effects of inhalational agents sensitising the myocardium to catecholamines and will pass off as the anaesthetic is eliminated.

If the irregularity persists or is accompanied by hypotension or poor peripheral perfusion, its nature should be established by ECG monitoring.

Although any type of dysrhythmia can occur post-operatively, premature atrial and ventricular contractions and atrial fibrillation are most commonly seen.

Premature Atrial Contractions (PACs)

A premature P wave is followed by a normal QRS complex (Fig. 4.7). This dysrhythmia usually causes no problems and no treatment is required.

Premature Ventricular Contractions (PVCs)

There is no P wave before a premature QRS complex. The complex is abnormally wide, notched or large and followed by a compensatory pause (Fig 4.8). If premature contractions follow each normal contraction, the term pulsus bigeminus is used.

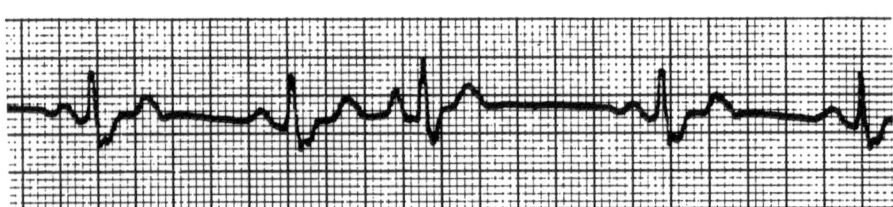

Fig. 4.7. Premature atrial contractions

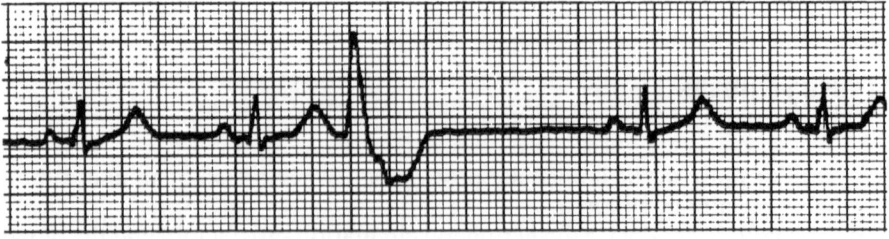

Fig. 4.8. Premature ventricular contractions

Causes

1. Hypoxia
2. Hypercarbia
3. Acidosis
4. Hypokalaemia
5. Digitalis overdose
6. Excess circulating catecholamines
7. Hyperthyroidism

Management

If the premature beats are infrequent and there is no accompanying hypotension, no treatment is required. If, however, they occur frequently (i.e. more than 5 per min), the underlying cause should be sought and corrected, since it may lead to ventricular tachycardia or ventricular fibrillation.

Treatment is by intravenous lignocaine (lidocaine) in a bolus of 1 mg/kg followed by an intravenous infusion at a rate of 1–4 mg/minute. Alternatively a β-blocker such as propranolol may be given in 1 mg increments.

Atrial Fibrillation

Absent P waves. Irregularly occuring QRS complexes (Fig. 4.9). Usually occurs as a result of a long-standing condition, e.g. mitral stenosis or coronary artery disease.

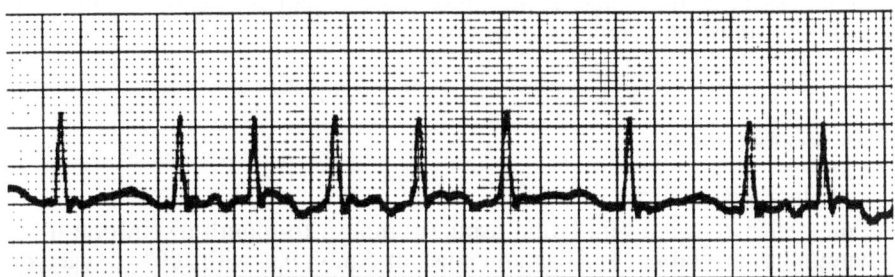

Fig. 4.9. Atrial fibrillation

Management

No treatment is required unless the ventricular response is rapid and the pulse rate exceeds 120 per minute or there are accompanying signs of heart failure or hypotension. The following should then be considered:

1. Cardioversion, using a synchronised D.C. shock
2. Digitalisation. This should not precede cardioversion, as the latter may precipitate a cardiac arrest in the digitalised patient

Many patients with atrial fibrillation are already digitalised prior to surgery so that neither cardioversion nor further digitalisation are appropriate. In this case a slow intravenous injection of disopyramide over 5 min to a total of 2 mg/kg or until the ventricular rate drops may be successful.

Cardiac Arrest

Cardiac arrest occurring in the recovery room should be treated vigorously and has every prospect of success because:

1. The precipitating cause is usually reversible, e.g. hypoxia, electrolyte imbalance, hypovolaemia
2. The patient is under continuous observation and there may be some advance warning, e.g. hypotension, cyanosis, bradycardia
3. Resuscitation equipment and trained staff are instantly available

The diagnosis is made when there is:

1. Loss of consciousness
2. No breathing
3. No pulse palpable in a major artery e.g. carotid or femoral artery

Examining the pupils, listening for heart sounds or connecting an ECG monitor are unnecessary at this stage. If no major pulse is palpable, cardiopulmonary resuscitation must be commenced without delay.

Initial Management

1. Establish a clear airway.
2. Commence artificial ventilation using (a) mouth-to-mouth respiration if no equipment available, (b) a bag and mask or Ambu bag with 100% oxygen or (c) intubation with cuffed tube as soon as possible. Give two large breaths ensuring that the lungs are seen to inflate.
3. Commence external cardiac massage by giving vigorous downwards thrusts on the lower third of the sternum with the palms of the hands at a rate of 80 per minute. After every 15 compressions of the heart, pause and give two inflations of the lungs. At this rate, there will be about 60 compressions of the heart each minute at a rate of 15 compressions to 2 inflations. This cycle must be continued until a spontaneous heartbeat is established.
4. Elevate foot of bed to improve venous return.

Subsequent Management

5. Establish an intravenous infusion if this is not already present so that all drugs can be given intravenously.
6. Montior ECG to establish the electrical activity of the heart. If ventricular fibrillation is shown (Fig. 4.10):

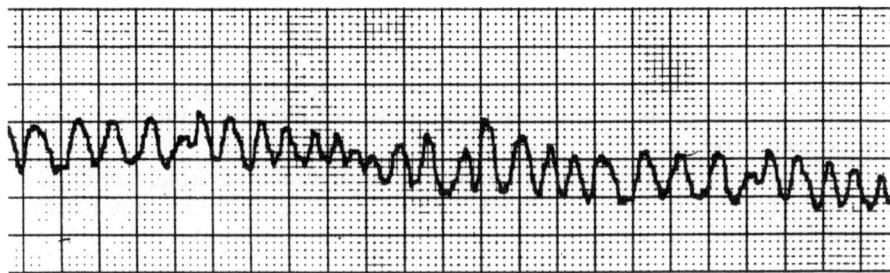

Fig. 4.10. Ventricular fibrillation

   a) Defibrillate heart using D.C. defibrillator with paddle placed across heart (Fig 4.11). Start with 200 joules. If no pulse is palpable immediately after the first shock, continue cardiac massage whilst the defibrillator is re-charged to 200 joules. Give a second shock.

   b) If defibrillation fails again, repeat cardiac massage (and ventilation) and then give a third shock of 400 joules.

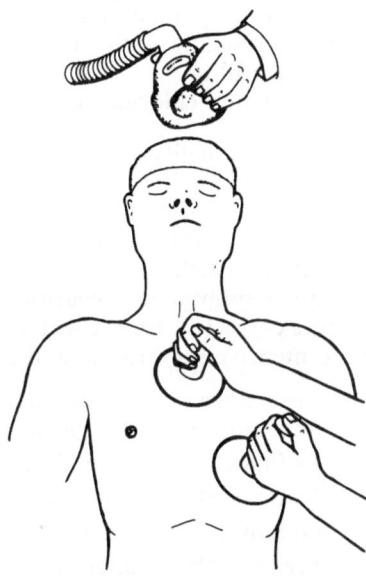

Fig. 4.11. Application of defibrillator paddles.
Assistants must stand well clear.

   c) If the third shock fails to establish a normal rhythm, give lignocaine 100 mg (10 ml 1% solution or 5 ml 2% solution) followed by a fourth shock of 400 joules.

   d) If unsuccessful, give adrenaline (epinephrine) 1 mg (10 ml 1:10 000 solution) followed by a fifth shock of 400 joules.

   e) If unsuccessful, give sodium bicarbonate 50 ml 8.4% solution and a sixth shock.

Ventilation and external cardiac massage should only be interrupted when a D.C. shock is about to be administered.

   In refractory ventricular fibrillation, bretylium 400 mg may be tried. It has a slow onset, so resuscitation should be continued even if it initially appears to be ineffective.

7. If, instead of ventricular fibrillation, the monitor shows asystole, ventilation and external cardiac massage should be performed as above and the following drugs administered:

   a) Atropine 1 mg

   b) Adrenaline (epinephrine) 1 mg (10 ml of 1 : 10 000 solution)

   c) Isoprenaline (isoproterenol) 100 μg

If they fail to produce ventricular fibrillation or a rhythm with a cardiac output, transvenous or oesophageal pacing should be considered.

8. There is a third mechanism of cardiac arrest: electro-mechanical dissociation. There may be normal or near-normal electrical activity shown on the monitor but it is not accompanied by any useful cardiac output. It has a poor prognosis.

   a) Consider and exclude mechanical causes such as cardiac tamponade or tension pneumothorax

   b) Adrenaline (epinephrine) 1 mg (10 ml of 1: 10 000 solution) may be helpful *or*

   c) Calcium chloride 10 ml of 10% solution

If there is difficulty in inserting an intravenous cannula in a collapsed patient, atropine, adrenaline and lignocaine can be given via the endotracheal tube. Absorption is rapid from the bronchial mucosa. Twice the intravenous dose is usually given. Intracardiac injections are hazardous, offer few advantages and are best avoided.

   Once a spontaneous heartbeat has been re-established and any precipitating factors corrected, the patient should be transferred to an intensive care unit so that intensive monitoring and further treatment can be given:

1. Ensure breathing is adequate. Consider a period of artificial ventilation. If a pneumothorax is suspected, insert a chest drain.

2. Estimate arterial blood gases: further bicarbonate may be necessary.

3. Estimate serum potassium.

4. Obtain a chest X-ray.

5. Measure the arterial blood pressure.

6. Insert a urinary catheter and monitor the urine output.
7. Insert a nasogastric tube and aspirate the stomach contents.
8. Insert a central venous catheter if indicated.
9. Obtain a 12-lead ECG.
10. Consider high-dose steroids to protect an ischaemic brain.

Miscellaneous Complications

Delayed Return of Consciousness

Most patients will have regained consciousness within 15 min of arrival in the recovery room. If unconsciousness persists for longer than 30 min a cause should be sought.

Causes

1. Drugs
   a) Relative overdose of drugs
      i) Excess administration, e.g. premedication, opiate supplements.
      ii) Increased sensitivity, e.g. in the elderly, cachectic or hypothyroid patient
      iii) Diminished metabolism, e.g. in liver dysfunction, hypothermia, hypothyroidism
   b) Drugs with prolonged action, e.g. ketamine, droperidol, lorazepam, repeat doses of barbiturates
2. Hypoglycaemia
3. Hypercarbia
4. Metabolic acidosis
5. Cerebral damage, which may result from a period of cerebral hypoxia or from a cerebrovascular accident during anaesthesia
6. Uraemia

Management

1. Ensure that the airway is clear and that respiration is adequate.
2. Reverse depression due to opiates with naloxone.
3. Check blood sugar. Treat hypoglycaemia with 50 ml of 50% glucose intravenously.

4. Check blood gases to exclude hypercarbia or metabolic acidosis. Treat with assisted ventilation or intravenous sodium bicarbonate as appropriate.
5. Consider flumazenil if benzodiazepines have been given.
6. Make a thorough examination of the central nervous system, taking a special note of localising signs, and record the findings as a baseline for future reference.
7. If there is still no response after 2–3 hours and the obvious causes have been treated, the patient should be transferred to an intensive care unit for subsequent management.

Restlessness, Excitement and Delirium

The immediate post-operative period may be accompanied by various degrees of excitement ranging from mild restlessness to violent uncontrolled movement.

Causes

1. Airway obstruction, especially caused by nasal packs (see p. 120)
2. Anxiety
3. Pain
4. Full bladder
5. Inadequate reversal of muscle relaxants
6. Cerebral hypoxia
7. Drugs. Elderly patients in particular can be extremely sensitive to drugs used in premedication, e.g. hyoscine, phenothiazines and barbiturates
8. Middle ear surgery. Restlessness is frequent following this type of surgery, possibly due to a temporary disturbance of the labyrinthine mechanism
9. Raised intracranial pressure
10. Hyperthyroidism
11. Psychological distress, e.g. following termination of pregnancy

Management

1. *Reassurance*. Anxious patients finding themselves in unfamiliar surroundings may become restless. They will frequently settle with gentle handling and sympathetic reassurance.
2. *Restraint*. Care must be taken to prevent the more vigorous patients injuring themselves. Cot sides should be raised. If it is necessary for patients to be restrained, minimal force should be used.

3. *Analgesics.* Administration should be intravenous, as required to relieve pain. Many patients will be unable to complain of pain in the immediate post-operative period. However, in the absence of other obvious causes, restlessness, especially if accompanied by tachycardia and hypertension, will usually respond to analgesic therapy.

4. *Give oxygen by face mask.*

5. *Ensure adequate reversal of relaxants,* giving further atropine and neostigmine if required. If ventilation remains inadequate, intubation and assisted ventilation may be needed.

6. *Reverse excessive premedication* due to above mentioned drugs by intravenous physostigmine 1–3 mg.

7. *Catheterise the bladder* if it is distended.

8. Following trauma or neurosurgery, raised intracranial pressure must always be considered, especially if the restlessness is accompanied by hypertension and bradycardia. If this is the case, a *neurological observation chart* should be begun at once and further advice sought.

Nausea and Vomiting

With improvements in anaesthetic drugs and techniques over the years, the incidence of post-operative vomiting has undoubtedly decreased. However, as one can never be absolutely certain that the stomach is empty even in fasted patients, recovery staff must be alert to the possibility of vomiting.

Causes

Various individual factors contribute to the incidence of post-operative vomiting. The results of numerous studies have shown it to be more frequent:

1. In those prone to motion sickness
2. In females rather than males
3. Following the use of ether or cyclopropane
4. With increasing duration of anaesthesia
5. Following the use of opiate medication. The effect is exacerbated with early mobilisation and reduced with the concurrent use of atropine, hyoscine or antihistamines
6. Following episodes of hypoxia or hypotension
7. Following intra-abdominal surgery
8. In the presence of severe pain
9. After middle ear surgery
10. Following the use of nitrous oxide

Management

Because of the danger of respiratory obstruction or aspiration resulting from vomiting, the recovery patient should be nursed on a tipping trolley and with suction apparatus to hand. Unless contraindicated (e.g. because of orthopaedic traction), the patient should normally be on his side to enable vomited material to be cleared from the pharynx by gravity. In the event of vomiting:

1. Tip head down
2. Suck out pharynx
3. Turn patient on to side if not already in this position (normally on left side in case subsequent laryngoscopy is required). This requires the help of an assistant.
4. If respiratory obstruction persists, clear the pharynx under direct vision using a laryngoscope
5. Give oxygen by mask

For treatment of aspiration of gastric contents, see p. 76

When vomiting or nausea persists for more than a brief period and pain can be excluded as a cause, anti-emetics such as prochlorperazine, metoclopramide or droperidol may be given intravenously or intramuscularly. The routine use of anti-emetics, however, is not recommended since persistent vomiting is not a problem in the majority of patients. Prophylactic anti-emetics are given:

1. Where vomiting is particularly undesirable, such as following a perforating eye injury, where it may cause a rise in intra-ocular pressure, or when the jaws have been wired together and suction is difficult
2. If there is a history of post-operative vomiting

   Following anti-emetic therapy, extra-pyramidal effects (e.g. muscle rigidity, restlessness, oculogyric crisis) have sometimes occurred, particularly after repeated doses of long-acting agents. These are very frightening to the patient and can be treated with anti-Parkinson-type drugs such as benzhexol or procyclidine.

Shivering

Shivering is frequently seen during recovery from general anaesthesia and may be so severe as to resemble grand mal epilepsy.

Causes

1. *Inhalational anaesthetic agents.* Shivering is commonest after the use of halothane but may follow other agents. The exact mechanism is unclear, although it has been shown to be unrelated to temperature change

2. *Blood transfusion reactions* (p. 101)
3. *Hypothermia* (p. 98).

Management

Although shivering is usually transient and does not often present a problem the following measures can be taken:

1. *Administration of oxygen* to increase F_1O_2. Shivering increases metabolic rate and so causes excess oxygen demand. Demand may exceed supply unless additional oxygen is administered.
2. *Extra blankets* if the patient is cold. Aluminium foil space blankets can be used if there is significant hypothermia.

Convulsions

Causes

1. *Cerebral irritation* due to:

   a) Trauma
   b) Neurosurgery
   c) A hypoxic episode
   d) Presence of intracranial mass
2. *Febrile convulsions*
   The combination of:

   a) Pre-operative pyrexia
   b) Dehydration
   c) Atropine medication, which reduces sweating
   d) Inhalational anaesthetics, which may interfere with the heat-regulating centre (especially diethyl ether)
   e) Excessive coverings, which may result in convulsions, especially in children
3. *Epilepsy*, particularly if anticonvulsant drugs have been omitted prior to surgery
4. *Drugs*
   a) Local anaesthetics: convulsions may result if the total quantity injected is excessive or if there has been an inadvertent intravascular injection. Special care is required when releasing a tourniquet following a Bier's block and when topping up an epidural in the recovery room in case the tip of the catheter has migrated into a vein

   b) Diethyl ether, especially in large doses accompanied by dehydration or fever

   c) Enflurane, especially in high concentrations with hyperventilation

   d) Methohexitone (methohexital)

5. *Eclampsia*
Preventative measures against convulsions must be continued into the post-operative period.

6. *Hypoglycaemia*

7. *Dilutional hyponatraemia*

8. *Uraemia*

Management

Regardless of the cause, oxygen is administered and convulsions terminated as rapidly as possible because of the dangers posed by an uncontrolled airway and excessive oxygen demand. Thiopentone (thiopental), diazepam, phenobarbitone (phenobarbital) and sodium valproate (valproic acid) are suitable drugs for this purpose. In extreme cases muscle relaxants, such as suxamethonium, (succinylcholine), intubation and artificial respiration may be needed. Once the convulsions have been controlled, attempts should be made to determine the underlying cause and to correct it.

Hypothermia

Agents used during general anaesthesia may depress the heat-regulating centre in the hypothalamus, causing vasodilatation or impaired shivering. Consequently some fall in temperature is not uncommon post-operatively, but with the use of thermostatically controlled operating theatres this is seldom severe except at the extremes of age.

Causes

1. Prolonged bowel exposure
2. Prolonged surgery in infants (because of their greater tendency to lose heat, see p. 137)
3. Intravenous infusions of large quantities of cold solutions or blood
4. Following deliberate hypothermia employed during cardiac or neurosurgery
5. Hypothyroidism
6. Bladder irrigation with cold fluids

Management

Hypothermia may lead to:

1. Myocardial depression or irritability
2. Metabolic acidosis
3. Altered response to neuromuscular blocking agents
4. Poor respiratory effort and hypoxia, particularly in children

If the temperature is low:

1. Prevent further heat loss by giving extra warmed blankets or wrapping the patient in an aluminium foil space blanket
2. Give intravenous fluids through a warming coil
3. In the case of infants the use of a warmed incubator or overhead heater is recommended
4. Monitor temperature. This should be done continuously if possible or at frequent intervals. The core temperature is a more valuable guide than skin temperature and this can be measured either with a nasopharyngeal, oesophageal or rectal probe. A low reading thermometer may be necessary in extreme cases
5. Keep patient in recovery unit until temperature has risen above 35 °C
6. In neonates hypothermia can interfere with respiratory effort. If this occurs, intubation and assisted ventilation may be required until normothermia has been achieved

Hyperthermia

A moderate rise in temperature (e.g. up to 39 °C) unaccompanied by other signs or symptoms does not in itself constitute a problem. However, the origin shoud be sought since it may require treatment in the recovery room.

Causes

1. *Infection*. This may have been present before surgery or may first become apparent immediately afterwards, especially following bowel or urological surgery
2. *Impaired heat loss*. The combination of pre-operative pyrexia, atropine (which reduces sweating), a high ambient temperature and the use of agents which interfere with the heat-regulating centre (especially diethyl ether) can cause hyperthermia, particularly in children
3. *Pyrogens* introduced during blood transfusion
4. *Malignant hyperpyrexia* (see below)

Management

1. Where infection is considered likely, appropriate antibiotic therapy may be commenced intravenously. If blood culture is contemplated, it should precede the administration of antibiotics.
2. If hyperthermia follows blood transfusion this should be stopped immediately and a sample of the transfused blood saved for analysis (p. 107).
3. Severe hyperpyrexia (>39°C), especially in children, will result in increased oxygen consumption and carbon dioxide production with metabolic and respiratory acidosis, causing increased demands on cardiac and respiratory function. This may result in cerebral hypoxia and convulsions and should be treated vigorously by:

   a) Active cooling with tepid sponging, ice and fans
   b) Oxygen therapy
   c) Intravenous diazepam as required to control convulsions.

Malignant Hyperthermia

This is a rare condition of unknown aetiology characterised by a rise in temperature of up to 1°C every 15 min which can be rapidly fatal unless treated immediately. It is often triggered off by anaesthesia and especially by the use of suxamethonium (succinylcholine) or halothane, although other anaesthetic agents and relaxants have been implicated. Evidence suggests that there is a hereditary defect in the calcium-storing membrane of the skeletal and cardiac muscle cells so that calcium is released into the cytoplasm with the production of heat.

The temperature rise may immediately follow after the triggering mechanism or there may be an interval of 30–45 min, so that it may not become obvious until the patient has reached the recovery room.

The family practitioner should be notified so that other members of the family may be screened for this abnormality.

Clinical features

1. Extreme pyrexia
2. Cyanosis
3. Tachycardia and tachypnoea
4. Metabolic and respiratory acidosis
5. Hyperkalaemia
6. Muscle rigidity (in 60% of patients)
7. Coagulopathy

Management

1. Hyperventilation with 100% oxygen
2. Vigorous cooling with ice and fans

3. Sodium bicarbonate to correct acidosis. (Monitoring of blood gases will be required)
4. Intravenous dextrose 20% and 10 units of soluble insulin to reduce hyper-kalaemia
5. Intravenous dantrolene 1 mg/kg every 5 min (up to 10 mg/kg may be required). Dantrolene inhibits the release of calcium into the muscle cell
6. Intravenous frusemide (furosemide) or mannitol to increase urinary output and prevent casts of myoglobin from blocking the renal tubules

Because of the rapidity of onset and the urgency of treatment, a malignant hyperthermia pack with all the necessary drugs should be readily available in the recovery room.

Blood Transfusion Reactions

Blood transfusion may be in progress when patients are admitted to the recovery room or alternatively it may become necessary during the immediate post-operative period. In either event, recovery staff must be alert for transfusion reactions which may be febrile, allergic or haemolytic. As patients are covered with drapes during surgery, skin reactions may only become obvious when these are removed at the end of the procedure.

Febrile Reactions

Febrile reactions occur in 1%–2% of transfusions and are generally caused by anti-leucocyte antibodies in the transfused blood. They are relatively slow in onset, the usual time from the start of transfusion being 2–4 h. Reactions may be more severe when blood is being transfused rapidly.

1. *Mild febrile reactions.* Temperature below 39 °C, no other symptoms or signs

   a) Slow the transfusion rate
   b) Administer antipyretics, e.g. paracetamol (acetaminophen)
2. *Severe febrile reactions.* Temperature above 39 °C, accompanied by rigors

   a) Stop transfusion
   b) Actively cool patient with tepid sponging and fans

   Bacterial contamination of transfused blood may initially present in this way. If this is suspected or there are accompanying signs of cardiovascular collapse:

   c) Give broad spectrum antibiotic
   d) Support the circulation by intravenous infusion
   e) Take appropriate blood samples and return the unit of blood and any previous units to the blood bank for bacteriological examination and serological testing

Allergic Reactions

1. *Mild.* Itching, rash
   a) Continue transfusion
   b) Administer antihistamines, e.g. chlorpheniramine 10 mg i.m.
2. *Severe.* Oedema, bronchospasm, hypotension
   a) Stop transfusion
   b) Support circulation by intravenous infusion
   c) Administer hydrocortisone 100 mg i.v.
   d) Consider adrenaline (epinephrine) 1 mg (1 ml 1:1000 solution) i.v.

Haemolytic Reactions

Haemolytic reactions are caused by incompatible blood transfusion. Haemo-
lysed red cells release free haemoglobin which can cause renal damage. Reactions are characterised by:

1. Localised pain   These signs are mask⎤ by
2. Loin or retrosternal pain   unconsciousness

3. Flushing
4. Pyrexia
5. Dyspnoea
6. Cardiovascular collapse
7. Oliguria
8. Haematuria

The picture may be complicated in 50% of patients by the development of
disseminated intravascular coagulation. If this occurs:

1. Stop transfusion and take down giving set
2. Support circulation by intravenous infusion
3. Give intravenous hydrocortisone 1 g
4. Send the unit of blood and any previously used packs together with a clotted
   sample of blood and anticoagulated samples for platelet count, clotting
   studies and examination for free Hb (p. 104)
5. Catheterise the bladder and monitor urine output. Send sample of urine for
   examination for Hb and urobilinogen
6. Stimulate urine production with frusemide (furosemide) or mannitol
7. Alkalinise urine with i.v. sodium bicarbonate to increase solubility of free Hb

Problems Associated with Massive Blood Transfusion

In addition to the normal hazards of any blood transfusion, whenever large volumes of blood have to be transfused rapidly (e.g. 500 ml every 5 min for 30 min), further problems may be anticipated as a result of changes in the stored blood.

Hypothermia

Since blood is normally stored at 4 °C the rapid infusion of cold blood will reduce body temperature and lead to:

1. Dysrhythmias and, in extreme cases, cardiac arrest
2. A shift of the oxygen dissociation curve to the left with impairment of oxygen release in the tissues

To eliminate these complications, large transfusions of blood should first pass through a blood warmer so that when it is transfused it is at body temperature.

Acidosis

Stored blood becomes progressively more acidostic and may have a pH of below 7.0. This is partly due to the presence of citrate in the anticoagulant and partly due to continuing anaerobic metabolism with lactic acid production. Since the shocked patient may already be acidotic, the resulting pH may become so low as to interfere with myocardial function and the reversal of muscle relaxants. This can be corrected by giving sodium bicarbonate intravenously, titrating the amount according to serial acid–base determinations. Bicarbonate should not, however, be given routinely as a metabolic alkalosis may result and further impair myocardial function.

Citrate Intoxication

Ionised calcium in stored blood is reduced by binding to citrate which is used as an anticoagulant. Under normal circumstances, the body has sufficient stores of calcium in the skeleton to compensate for this. However, following a massive transfusion or when citrate metabolism is impaired by liver disease, hypocalcaemia may result. This causes myocardial depression and hypotension. On the ECG, the ST segment is prolonged.

The treatment is to give 10 ml of 10% calcium gluconate slowly until the hypotension and ECG abnormalities are corrected.

Hyperkalaemia

Potassium diffuses from red cells during storage at a rate approaching 1 mmol per day so that at the end of 28 days' storage, blood may contain up to 30 mmol per litre. This may lead to significant hyperkalaemia (especially if renal function is impaired) with high peaked T waves on ECG and cardiac irritability. These effects can be countered by giving calcium gluconate, as described above. Alternatively, as insulin causes potassium to move intracellularly, 10 units of soluble insulin and 20 ml 50% dextrose can be given.

Micro-emboli

Stored blood contains micro-aggregates consisting of cell remnants and threads of fibrin ranging in diameter from 20 to 200 μm. Following transfusion these are filtered by the microcirculation in the lungs and lead to the development of adult respiratory distress syndrome (ARDS). This effect can be minimised by passing blood through a microfilter of pore size 20–40 μm and this is recommended for transfusions exceeding 1 litre. The resulting increased resistance can be overcome by using a pressure bag to maintain flow.

Failure of Coagulation (see below)

Stored blood rapidly becomes deficient in clotting factors (especially V, VII, and VIII) and platelets so that following a massive transfusion, their levels may become significantly reduced. These deficiencies can normally be made good with fresh frozen plasma, one unit for every five units of blood, and platelet concentrate, one unit for every ten units of blood. Coagulation studies will be required if bleeding persists despite this regime.

Failure of Coagulation

Persistent bleeding in the immediate post-operative period may be due to defective coagulation. Damage to blood vessels results in an accumulation of platelets around which fibrin clot is formed. A variety of clotting factors must be present in the blood to allow the conversion of fibrogen into the fibrin filaments:

    I Fibrinogen
   II Prothrombin
  III Thromboplastin
  IV Calcium
   V Pro-accelerin
  VI Not allocated
 VII Pro-convertin

VIII Anti-haemophilic factor
  IX Christmas factor
   X Stuart-Power factor
  XI Plasma thromboplastin antecedent
 XII Hageman factor
XIII Fibrin stabilising factor

The fibrin clot is eventually lysed by plasmin, which is formed by conversion of the inactive plasminogen.

Causes

1. *Congenital deficiency of clotting factors.* Normally a single factor is deficient, e.g. haemophilia A (factor VIII) or Christmas disease (factor IX). This is usually recognised prior to surgery and the deficient factor is replaced pre- and post-operatively. This requires frequent assays of the appropriate factor. Formerly, some preparations of these factors were contaminated with the AIDS virus and many haemophiliacs were infected. The preparations currently used carry no risk.

2. *Massive blood transfusion.* Stored blood rapidly becomes deficient in clotting factors (especially V, VII and VIII) and subsequently in platelets. In addition, calcium is bound by the citrate anticoagulant and the resulting hypocalcaemia may contribute to deficient coagulation.

3. *Anticoagulants*
   a) *Heparin* acts at several sites in the coagulation process. It is frequently given intravenously during cardiovascular surgery and may be reversed by protamine sulphate. Care must be taken with protamine treatment since excess amounts may also act as an anticoagulant.
   b) *Coumarin-type drugs*, e.g. warfarin sodium. These inhibit the vitamin K-dependent carboxylation of clotting factors II, VII, IX and X in the liver. Rapid reversal cannot, therefore, be achieved by simply giving intravenous vitamin K_1 preparations such as phytomenadione (phytonadione) as fresh clotting factors have to be synthesised in the liver. If rapid reversal of anti-coagulation is required, fresh frozen plasma should be given.

4. *Liver disease.* Most clotting factors are synthesised in the liver and may be deficient in severe liver dysfunction.

5. *Vitamin K deficiency.* Vitamin K absorption is impaired in obstructive jaundice and following pre-operative bowel sterilisation with anitbiotics.

6. *Disseminated intravascular coagulation (DIC).* In the following clinical states there is massive deposition of fibrin throughout the microcirculation, resulting in the consumption of clotting factors and platelets with consequent bleeding:

   a) Prolonged shock with tissue hypoxia
   b) Extensive tissue damage, e.g. trauma, burns, prolonged surgery

c) Infection, e.g. acute viral infection, septicaemia
d) Obstetric emergencies, e.g. amiotic fluid embolism, intrauterine death, abruptio placentae, toxaemia
e) Acute haemolysis, e.g. mismatched transfusion
f) Following prostatectomy
g) Extracorporeal circulation

Extensive fibrinolysis follows, with the liberation of fibrin degradation products and thence further bleeding. The condition is therefore characterised by clotting and bleeding occurring simultaneously.

7. *Thrombocytopenia* (platelet deficiency). Platelets are not only required to initiate haemostasis by plugging damaged blood vessels but are also essential in the coagulation process. If the platelet count falls below 50×10^9/litre, a failure of coagulation may occur.

Causes of thrombocytopenia seen post-operatively:

a) *Dilution of platelets.* Transfusion of stored blood deficient in platelets leads to a reduction in circulating platelet count. This reduction is more than can be accounted for by dilution alone. Significant reduction in platelet count is often observed after the rapid transfusion of six or more units of stored blood.
b) *Depressed platelet formation*, e.g. as seen in patients with leukaemia, cancer, uraemia and during chemotherapy.
c) *Excessive utilisation of platelets*, e.g. in disseminated intravascular coagulation.
d) *Idiopathic thrombocytopenia.* A rare condition of unknown aetiology seen mainly in young adults and characterised by purpura and petechiae.
e) *Excessive destruction of platelets*, e.g. in hypersplenism.

Management

To determine the cause of a failure of coagulation will require a series of laboratory tests:

1. *Platelet count* (EDTA bottle). Normal values $150–400 \times 10^9$/litre. Bleeding is unusual if the value is above 50×10^9/litre.
2. *Prothrombin time* (sodium citrate bottle). Normal value, approximately 12 s. Therapeutic ratio is 2–4 times the normal value. Prolonged in deficiency of factors II, V, VIII and X, e.g. as seen in liver disease, vitamin K deficiency, anticoagulant therapy and DIC.
3. *Activated partial thromboplastin time* (APTT) (sodium citrate bottle); also kaolin cephalin clotting time (KCCT). Normal values, 25–40 s. Prolonged in deficiency of factors II, V, VIII, IX, X, XI, and XII e.g. as seen in anticoagulant therapy, haemophilia A, Christmas disease.
4. *Fibrin degradation products* (FDPs) (bottle with soya bean trypsin inhibitor). Normal values $< 10\mu g$/ml. Raised in DIC. (Smaller rises are found following major surgery, trauma, deep vein thrombosis and pulmonary embolism.

5. *Fibrinogen level* (sodium citrate bottle). In this test the plasma is diluted to give the titre, i.e. the greater the fibrinogen content the more the dilution. Normal values $> 1 : 64$; Low values, $< 1 : 64$. The test may be modified to detect the presence of a circulating inhibitor or fibrinolysins. Fibrinogen is deficient in liver disease, in DIC and after massive blood transfusion.

6. *Thrombin clotting time* (TCT) (sodium citrate bottle). Normal values, 20–30 s. Prolonged when fibrinogen is deficient or abnormal and in the presence of inhibitory substances, e.g. FDPs, heparin.

The above tests are not, however, necessary for rational therapy to be given; the immediate history will usually supply sufficient information for this purpose.

1. *Following major transfusion of stored blood* it can be predicted that clotting factors, platelets and available calcium will be reduced. This can be corrected by the administration of:

   a) Fresh frozen plasma. This contains all the clotting factors and can normally be made available within 20 min. Adequate levels can be maintained by giving one unit of fresh frozen plasma for every five units of blood.

   b) Platelet concentrate. This has to be specially prepared at a transfusion centre from freshly donated blood. As it deteriorates rapidly it should be used without delay. A blood filter should not be used for the infusion of platelets.

   c) Intravenous calcium gluconate 10%. Increments of 10 ml may be needed for every litre of blood if it is being transfused rapidly. This is mainly to counter myocardial depression due to hypocalcaemia, which only rarely interferes with coagulation.

2. *Following cardiovascular surgery* persistent heparinisation may require reversal by intravenous protamine sulphate. In calculating dosage, allowance should be made for the metabolism of heparin, and protamine given in minimal amounts since excess protamine itself interferes with coagulation.

If these simple measures do not correct the situation and the clinical picture suggests the possibility of disseminated intravascular coagulation, further action is urgently required:

1. *Consult a haematologist.* It is wise to enlist the help of an experienced haematologist at an early stage since inappropriate therapy will not only waste valuable time but make subsequent management more difficult.

2. *Draw blood for coagulation tests.* As the coagulation profile may be constantly changing it is important that all the blood required for the various tests is taken at the same time.

3. *Continue to replace blood* with the addition of fresh frozen plasma, platelets and calcium as required to prevent further deficiencies.

In the event of DIC being diagnosed, subsequent treatment will be aimed at:

1. Removal of precipitating stimulus is possible, e.g. evacuation of uterine contents,

2. Replacement of coagulation factors and, possibly,
3. Heparinisation — despite persistent bleeding this may be necessary to prevent continued intravascular coagulation with consumption of clotting factors.

Oliguria

Causes

Inadequate urine output (less than 0.5 ml/(kg·h)) may be due to the following causes:

1. *Pre-renal.* Inadequate renal perfusion due to hypovolaemia or hypotension, e.g. systolic readings of below 60 mmHg.
2. *Renal damage* due to:
   a) Sepsis
   b) Haemolysis
   c) Hypoxaemia
   d) Hypotension
   e) Antibiotic therapy, e.g. gentamicin
   f) Release of myoglobin, e.g. following crush injury, malignant hyperthermia
3. *Post-renal outflow obstruction*

The urine output is monitored post-operatively in patients at risk of developing acute renal failure. Indications include:

1. Impaired renal or cardiac function pre-operatively
2. Obstructive jaundice (see p. 150)
3. Episodes of hypoxia or hypotension
4. Cardiac or aortic surgery
5. Major trauma or severe blood loss
6. Septicaemia
7. Extensive burns
8. Crush injury
9. Mismatched transfusion
10. Pancreatitis
11. Malignant hyperthermia

Management

1. Exclude mechanical obstruction of urinary catheter caused by clots of blood or kinking. Bladder distension will suggest this. Change catheter if obstruction cannot be cleared.

2. Consider hypotension or hypovolaemia as the most likely causes. Measure the CVP, if necessary.
3. Infuse 250–500 ml of sodium chloride 0.9% intravenously. A subsequent increase in urine output confirms hypovolaemia, which must be corrected.

If these measures are unsuccessful and the urine production remains below 0.5 ml/(kg·h), acute renal failure may be imminent.

4. Urinary production may be stimulated by:

   a) mannitol 100 ml of 20% over 15 min
   b) frusemide (furosemide) 20–40 mg
   c) low dose dopamine infusion, i.e. up to 5 μg/(kg·min).

If an adequate renal output is not established following these measures, acute renal failure must be assumed to have occurred and the advice of a nephrologist should be sought as soon as possible. While the patient remains in the recovery unit it is important not to overload the circulation.

Further Reading

Andersen R, Krohg K (1976) Pain as a major cause of post-operative nausea. Can Anaesth Soc 23: 366–369

Asbury AJ (1981) Problems of the immediate post-anaesthesia period. Br J Hosp Med 25: 159–163

Barbour CM, Little DM (1957) Postoperative hypotension. JAMA 165: 1529–1532

Bay J, Nunn JF, Prys-Roberts C (1968) Factors influencing arterial Po_2 during recovery from anaesthesia. Br J Anaesth 40: 398–407

Bevan DR (1979) Renal function in anaesthesia and surgery. Academic Press, London

Buckley JJ, Jackson JA (1961) Postoperative cardiac arrhythmias. Anaesthesiology 22: 723–737

Cullen DJ, Cullen BL (1975) Postanaesthetic complications. Surg Clin North Am 55: 987–998

Darbyshire P (1988) C. V. P. monitoring. Nursing Times 24: 6, 36–38

Drain CB, Shipley SB (1979) Recovery room. WB Saunders, Philadelphia

Evans TR (ed) (1986) ABC of resuscitation. BMJ publications, London

Farman JV (1978) The work of the recovery room. Br J Hosp Med 19: 606–616

Farman JV, Hudson RBS, Andrewes S, Eltringham RJ (1979) Symposium: Recovery from anaesthesia. J R Soc Med 72: 270–280

Feeley TW (1980) The recovery room. In: Miller R D (ed) Anaesthesia, Churchill Livingstone, Edinburgh, New York

Gal TJ, Cooperman LH (1975) Hypertension in the immediate post-operative period, Br J Anaesth 47: 70–74

Gold MI (1969) Post-anaesthetic vomiting in the recovery room. Br J Anaesth 41: 143–149

Greenwalt TJ (ed) (1988) Blood transfusion. American Medical Association, Wisconsin

Hanson GC, Wright PL (eds)(1978) The medical management of the critically ill. Academic Press, London, Grune and Stratton, New York

Hinds CJ (1982) Current management of patients after cardiopulmonary bypass. Anaesthesia 37: 170–191

Jones RM, Hantler CB, Knight PR (1981) Use of pentolinium in post-operative hypertension resistant to sodium nitroprusside. Br J Anaesth 53: 1151–1154

Marshall BE, Wyche MQ (1972) Hypoxaemia during and after anaesthesia, Anaesthesiology 37: 178–209

Parkhouse J, Lambrechts W, Simpson BRJ (1961) The incidence of post-operative pain. Br J
    Anaesth 33: 345–353
Seeley HF (1978) The clinical management of the aspiration of gastric contents. J Int Med Res 6
    [Suppl 1]: 63–69
Stoddart JC (1978) Postoperative respiratory failure: An anaesthetic hazard? Br J Anaesth 50:
    695–700
White DC (1982) The relief of postoperative pain. In:Atkinson RS, Hewer C L (eds) Recent adv
    anaesth analg 14, Churchill Livingstone, Edinburgh, pp 121–139
Wynne JW, Modell JH (1977) Respiratory aspiration of stomach contents. Ann Intern Med 87:
    466–474

Chapter 5

Recovery in Different Branches of Surgery

Emergency Surgery

Many patients will present for emergency surgery without time for adequate pre-operative preparation. In some cases, history taking will have been inadequate and previous records may be unavailable. In these circumstances, potentially dangerous situations may surface for the first time during the recovery period.

Surgery for Trauma

1. *Full stomach.* Patients requiring emergency surgery following trauma must be assumed to have a full stomach. Efforts to empty the stomach before or during surgery by passing a nasogastric tube or administering metoclopramide are not invariably successful, so these patients should be nursed on their side with a slight head-down tilt. Extubation should be delayed until consciousness has returned and the patient objects to the presence of the tube. Vomiting may be copious and powerful suction with wide-bore tubing must be close at hand.

2. *Head injury.* A delayed return of consciousness may be due to alcohol, hypoglycaemia or head injury. If the history suggests the possibility of a head injury, regular neurological assessment using the Glasgow coma scale (see p. 126) is recommended.

   Opiate administration should be avoided if possible as it will:

   a) Depress the level of consciousness
   b) Depress respiration
   c) Interfere with examination of the pupils by causing constriction

Codeine phosphate is a suitable alternative without these disadvantages. If pain is inadequately controlled by codeine phosphate and more potent opiates are considered necessary, they should be administered intravenously in small increments until the minimal effective dose has been given.

3. *Associated injuries* may complicate the presenting surgical problem, for example:

   a) Fractured ribs and the possibility of pneumothorax or haemothorax (p. 78). Recovery staff must be alert to the possibility of tension pneumothorax (p. 79) developing rapidly, especially if intermittent positive pressure ventilation is being used.
   b) Ruptured spleen causing persistent hypovolaemia
   c) Fractured pelvis causing haematuria or anuria

4. *Hypovolaemia.* Blood loss is frequently underestimated following trauma, particularly if there have been large scalp wounds or fractures of the long bones or pelvis. If signs of hypovolaemia develop post-operatively (i.e. pallor, collapsed veins, weak thready pulse, increasing heart rate, decreasing blood pressure and oliguria), intravenous fluid replacement must be accelerated using, if necessary, CVP measurements to guide therapy.

Surgery in the Accident Department

The patient must be assumed to have a full stomach and recover from anaesthesia in the lateral position with head-down tilt and suction to hand.

Following recovery from general anaesthesia, the patient must remain under observation in the accident department for at least 2 h, during which time, recovery staff must satisfy themselves that the patient is fully conscious, that his movements are co-ordinated and that he is to be escorted home by a responsible adult. Patients who have been intubated are only allowed home provided there has been no evidence of laryngeal stridor in the 2 h following extubation. If suxamethonium (succinylcholine) has been used, the patient should be advised to restrict activity during the following 24 h to minimise muscle pains. The dangers of taking alcohol, driving, cooking or operating machinery during the next 24 h must be stressed, preferably in writing. An adequate supply of analgesics should be provided if post-operative pain is likely.

Gastroenterology

Endoscopy

The incidence of perforation of the oesophagus is negligible with the use of the fibre-optic endoscope. However, patients may be at risk of gastro-oesophageal reflux and aspiration into the lungs if they have a hiatus hernia and an incompetent cardia; thus it is particularly important that they are kept on their side while recovering from anaesthesia. When an oesophageal stricture is bypassed by the insertion of a tube, e.g. the Celestin tube, regurgitation of stomach contents becomes more likely and recovery staff should identify these patients at risk.

Perforation of the oesophagus is more likely when a rigid oesophagoscope has been used and after the dilatation of strictures (particularly those which are malignant), and it may first become evident in the recovery room.

The patient may complain of pain in the chest, neck or epigastrium. If they also develop pyrexia, tachycardia, hypotension and subcutaneous emphysema, it is probable that the oesophagus has been perforated. An intravenous infusion should be started and a chest X-ray taken while definitive management is arranged. The patient must not be allowed oral fluids.

Upper Gastrointestinal Tract Bleeding

Following operations to arrest bleeding, problems may occur in the recovery period because:

1. Blood replacement may have been inadequate
2. Complications of massive transfusion may arise (p. 103)
3. Further bleeding may occur. This may be either revealed (haematemesis, fresh blood draining from the nasogastric tube) or concealed. If signs of hypovolaemia (p. 80) persist despite blood replacement, the surgeon must be informed without delay.

If surgery has been performed because of bleeding from oesophageal varices (e.g. porto-caval anastamosis or oesophageal transection), problems associated with liver dysfunction (p. 150) may occur.

Surgery for Intestinal Obstruction or Peritonitis

Patients with these conditions can develop severe fluid and electrolyte disturbances which may not have been corrected by the time they reach the recovery unit. Hypovolaemia, hypokalaemia and metabolic acidosis are not uncommonly found and lead to poor peripheral perfusion, cardiovascular collapse, dysrhythmias and difficulty in reversing muscle relaxants. These problems are more dangerous in children, in whom fluid depletion is easily underestimated. The state of the peripheral circulation and measurements of central venous pressure, urine output, urea and electrolytes, together with blood gas analysis will provide useful guides for the correction of these abnormalities.

Bowel Surgery

Neostigmine is sometimes avoided following bowel surgery because of the damage it may cause to anastomoses by stimulating gut contraction. In such patients elective post-operative ventilation is continued until the effects of muscle relaxants have been eliminated.

Other problems occasionally encountered following bowel surgery include:

1. *Hypokalaemia* following prolonged diarrhoea or vigorous bowel wash-out. This may cause difficulty with reversal of muscle relaxants or dysrhythmias. Intravenous potassium supplements may be required.
2. *Hypothermia* following prolonged bowel exposure (see p. 98).
3. *Adrenocortical insufficiency* may develop in patients receiving prolonged steroid therapy for inflammatory diseases of the bowel (see p. 144).
4. *Septicaemia* (see p. 82) may occur with toxic megacolon seen in ulcerative colitis or following gall bladder surgery.
5. *Prolongation of muscle relaxants* owing to the administration of antibiotics (see p. 79).

Orthopaedic Surgery

Plaster Casts

When handling freshly applied plaster of Paris the palms of the hands should be used rather than the fingers, as they may cause indentations and subsequent discomfort. The principles of plaster cast care will also apply to compression bandages. The limb should be elevated to aid venous drainage and to reduce any consequent swelling. It should be supported on a firm pillow until the cast is fully hardened. One or more fingers or toes should be exposed so that any of the following signs of circulatory impairment can be readily observed:

1. Blanching of skin
2. Cyanosis — refer to normal limb for comparison
3. Prolonged circulatory filling time — assess after a brief period of compression with the fingers.
4. Fall in temperature
5. Sensory impairment

The cast margin should be checked to ensure that this is not causing undue pressure on the underlying tissues. This is of particular importance with lower limb casts which may cause a local pressure injury to the lateral popliteal nerve as it crosses the neck of the fibula. Pressure on this nerve will cause foot drop. It is important to note possible unprotected bony prominences which may be present. Bleeding should be noted and outlined on the plaster, together with the exact time of marking. If any untoward signs are present, the orthopaedic surgeon should be notified without delay.

Plaster jackets enclosing the thorax can restrict respirations. Adequate respiratory function must be confirmed before the patient is allowed to leave the recovery unit.

Traction

Traction cannot be adequately applied using the standard recovery trolley. If it is essential to apply traction in the immediate post-operative period the patient's own bed can be brought from the ward for this purpose. When heavy weights are used, elevation of the foot of the bed will be necessary.

Reduction of Fractures

When fractures have been manipulated, careful observation of the limb distal to the fracture is required so that vascular (see above) or neurological impairment will be swiftly identified.

Limbs and joints must be adequately supported in a comfortable position and signs of persistent blood loss on dressings or plasters, in drainage bottles or by increasing limb girth must be identified. If blood loss is significant, it may need to be replaced.

Hip Operations

Hip operations such as pin and plating are frequently performed on the frail and elderly, who may present with associated conditions, e.g. dehydration, anaemia, chest infection. Blood loss can be heavy and close observation of the cardio-vascular system is required. Further fluid replacement or blood transfusion may be required. Central venous pressure measurements are a useful guide to transfusion requirements in patients with cardiac failure. Spinal and epidural anaesthesia are often used to reduce blood loss but additional precautions are needed post-operatively following these techniques (pp. 59, 60 and 142).

The groin should be inspected to identify any damage to the vulva or scrotum caused by the central peg during surgery, and any extraneous plaster should be removed.

Because these patients frequently have atrophic skin, the rough canvas should be removed early and carefully from beneath them to avoid skin damage. Early transfer of these patients to their own bed in the recovery room is preferable to nursing them on firm trolleys.

Deep vein thrombosis is common and increases the risk of subsequent pulmonary embolism; early mobilisation and physiotherapy are employed to prevent venous stasis and reduce the risk of these complications.

Following hip replacement, steps must be taken to prevent dislocation. This may be done by using an abduction (Charnley) pillow. A patient who remains in the recovery unit for several hours should be turned on to the operated side to take pressure off the sacrum.

Fractured Vertebrae

Unstable vertebral fractures may cause damage to the spinal cord unless extreme caution is exercised when the patient is moved. Flexion, extension and twisting movements of the spine must be avoided and any lifting of the patient must be undertaken gently, slowly and in a co-ordinated way, with the vertebrae supported along their entire length either by a firm canvas or by an adequate number of assistants.

Fractures of the cervical vertebrae are generally stabilised by traction applied to skull calipers. When these patients have to be lifted, the anaesthetist's full attention will be required to ensure that the head and neck move as one with the rest of the body. As the patients cannot be turned on to their side in an emergency, extra care will be needed in keeping the airway clear, and observations must not be relaxed till the patient is fully conscious and able to protect his own airway.

Obstetrics and Gynaecology

Caesarean Section

There is a risk of inhaling gastric contents post-operatively until an effective cough reflex has returned. When surgery has been completed, the patient remains intubated and is nursed on her side with a head-down tilt until consciousness has returned and she starts to object to the presence of the tube. Only when the patient has demonstrated that she can protect her own airway can extubation be safely performed. The attendant should be able to tell the mother the sex and condition of her baby when asked.

When spinal or epidural anaesthesia has been used, a degree of residual motor, sensory and autonomic block must be expected post-operatively (p. 142).

Post-operative complications include:

1. *Post-partum haemorrhage:* The perineal pad is inspected regularly for signs of blood loss and the fundal height and degree of contraction checked. Fundal massage and the administration of oxytocics may be required. Oxytocin may be preferred in the presence of hypertension since ergometrine can itself cause a further rise in blood pressure. When oxytocin is used, a continuous infusion may be needed because of its short duration of action. Blood replacement will be required if there is continued loss. It might also be wise to take blood samples for coagulation studies (p. 104).

2. *Pre-eclamptic toxaemia.* Intense observations must be maintained post-operatively in patients with pre-eclamptic toxaemia as the signs of deterioration (increasing blood pressure, proteinuria, oedema and oliguria) must be detected and treated if convulsions are to be avoided (p. 97).
   Management includes:

   a) Avoidance of undue stimulation. It is preferable to transfer patients to a quiet, darkened room.

b) Sedation with a continuous infusion of diazepam or chlormethiazole in addition to analgesics.
c) Reduction of blood pressure, e.g. by an infusion of hydralazine titrated against the patient's response.
d) Fluid restriction.
e) Diuretics.

3. *Amniotic fluid embolism*. This rare condition may follow caesarean section or normal delivery and is characterised by a sudden onset of respiratory insufficiency and cardiovascular collapse. There is persistent bleeding with defective coagulation due to disseminated intravascular coagulation (p. 104).

Treatment consists of cardiovascular and respiratory support. Blood samples are taken for coagulation studies and the appropriate replacement therapy is given under the guidance of an experienced haematologist.

Evacuation of Retained Products of Conception; Suction Termination of Pregnancy

Perineal pads should be checked regularly for signs of continued bleeding. Further ergometrine or oxytocin should be given if required and hypovolaemia prevented by intravenous fluids or blood, if necessary.

A careful, understanding approach is needed for all patients after termination of pregnancy as emotional distress is common.

A perforated uterus must be suspected if there is:

1. Increasing pulse rate
2. Decreasing blood pressure
3. Pallor
4. Inappropriate abdominal pain

The surgeon must be informed without delay.

Laparoscopy

During this operation large volumes of carbon dioxide are insufflated into the peritoneal cavity. Although much of this is released at the end of the procedure, the abdomen may remain distended and pain and restlessness are common. Early administration of analgesics may be required.

Hysterectomy

Post-operative haemorrhage may complicate this operation so that close observation of the cardiovascular system and regular inspection of the wound dressing or pad must be undertaken. Vaginal packing may be required. If the ligature on the uterine pedicle slips, haemorrhage may be brisk and adequate blood replacement is required before further surgery.

When regional anaesthesia has been used, post-operative hypotension may occur but, provided peripheral perfusion is adequate and hypovolaemia is avoided, the blood pressure may be allowed to rise slowly as sympathetic tone returns (p. 142).

Ear, Nose and Throat Surgery

Tonsillectomy

Following surgery, patients are placed in the 'tonsil position' to allow optimal drainage of blood and secretions. The patient is turned well over on to one side with a pillow under the lower shoulder and the head down (see Fig. 5.1). An oral airway is inserted until the patient is conscious.

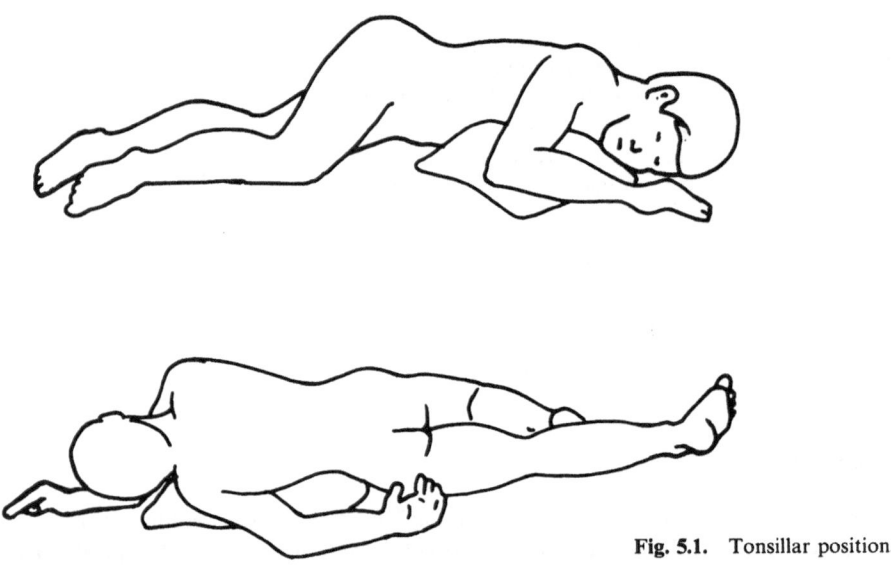

Fig. 5.1. Tonsillar position.

Blind suction is avoided, if possible as it may disturb clots of blood or displace ligatures, and cause further haemorrhage.

Post-operative haemorrhage is a serious complication which may rapidly lead to hypovolaemia if it is not detected early. It must be remembered that visible haemorrhage may represent only a small percentage of the blood lost, since much of the blood will be swallowed. Signs of persistent haemorrhage include:

1. Increased drainage of blood from the mouth
2. Coughing and spitting of blood

3. Frequent swallowing, sometimes followed by vomiting of blood
4. Pallor
5. Poor peripheral perfusion
6. Increasing pulse rate
7. Falling blood pressure

If these signs occur, blood should be taken for cross matching, an intravenous infusion established and the surgeon and anaesthetist informed without delay as further surgery may be required.

Laryngoscopy

The patient should be closely observed until the gag or cough reflexes return. The 'tonsil position' is used until the patient is fully conscious. If a local anaesthetic has been applied topically during this procedure, the patient should not be allowed oral fluids for 4 h. Recovery may be accompanied by:

1. Violent coughing and dyspnoea
2. Laryngospasm
3. Stridor
4. Bleeding, especially if a biopsy has been performed

Humidified oxygen and resting the voice may help minimise problems. If stridor is marked, the patient should be given a helium : oxygen mixture (80% helium : 20% oxygen) to breathe. This will reduce the work of breathing, relieve the patient's anxiety and frequently allow the stridor to disappear.

Tracheostomy

The recovery room staff should be forewarned of the arrival of any patient who has had a tracheostomy and should know the reason why the operation was necessary. The following should be readily available:

1. A range of tracheostomy tubes and a tracheal dilator
2. Adequate suction
3. Ambu bag
4. Suitable catheter mounts
5. Tracheostomy oxygen mask

Immediate complications of tracheostomy may include:

1. *Obstruction of the tube* by blood or secretions. Suctioning should be carried out in a sterile manner using a disposable soft suction catheter with an air control port. Viscide secretions can be reduced by humidifying the inspired air or oxygen since the normal humidifying mechanisms of the upper airway have been bypassed (see p. 36).

2. *Displacement of the tube.* The tracheostomy tube is secured in theatre using a double tie with reef knots. It should be sufficiently tight so that two fingers may just be inserted under the tape. If it is too loose, the tube may be expelled by coughing. This is a potential disaster as the tissue planes may move relative to one another. It can then be very difficult or impossible to replace the tracheostomy tube. After the tube has been in place for several days, a sinus forms. Removing and changing the tube is then relatively easy.

3. *Bleeding around wound edges*, which may require dressing changes.

Constant reassurance by recovery staff will be required as patients who have undergone tracheostomy may be very frightened and are unable to speak. Questions should be worded accordingly.

Operations on the Nose

Until fully conscious, these patients should remain in the tonsil position to allow free drainage of blood and mucosal fluid (see Fig. 5.1). Once consciousness has been regained, the semi-Fowler's position (Fig. 5.2) can be adopted to improve venous drainage and decrease local oedema.

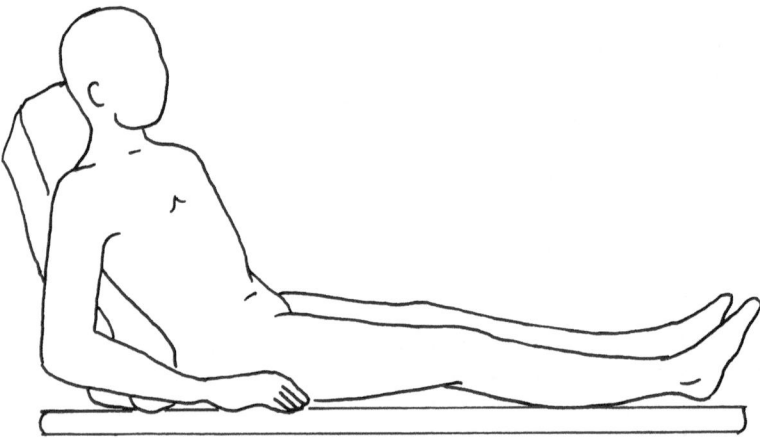

Fig. 5.2. Semi-Fowler's position.

A nasal pack is frequently inserted and held in place by taping it to the external nares. Its position should be checked and the amount of drainage noted. It is important that the pack should remain in this position as any movement into the post-nasal space may lead to subsequent airway obstruction.

Close observation must be maintained for signs of continued blood loss, much of which may trickle down the posterior pharyngeal wall and be swallowed (see 'Tonsillectomy', p. 118).

These patients sometimes become confused and delirious post-operatively, possibly because of feelings of panic due to nasal obstruction. They may forget to mouth breathe and try to remove the packs by every means they can. They should be reminded to breathe through the mouth and gently reassured. A Guedel airway may be a useful means of keeping the mouth open during this phase (p. 94).

When plaster of Paris has been applied to the nose following the reduction of fractured nasal bones, care must be taken to ensure that the patient does not roll over on to the nose and distort or displace the splint.

Hypotensive anaesthesia is frequently used for rhinoplasty. A degree of residual hypotension may persist into the post-operative period. Provided peripheral perfusion is adequate and hypovolaemia is avoided, blood pressure is allowed to rise slowly as the hypotensive agents are eliminated (p. 143).

Middle Ear Surgery

Hypotensive techniques are frequently employed for middle ear surgery and the post-operative nursing care is as outlined on p. 143.

A pressure bandage is usually applied at the end of surgery. The patient lies on the unoperated side and the dressing is inspected frequently for signs of bleeding. This can be a problem if the blood pressure is allowed to rise too quickly after hypotensive anaesthesia.

Restlessness and vertigo frequently occur, particularly if there has been direct vestibular stimulation. These may be worse if the patient sits up. The patient is encouraged to remain quiet and still and lie with a single pillow. Anti-emetics should be given. This is the rule for all recovering patients.

As the facial nerve may be damaged during surgery, its integrity should be confirmed by checking that there is full movement of the facial muscles. This may be done by asking the patient to show their teeth or smile.

Thyroid Surgery

Airway Problems

Airway problems may be caused by:

1. *Obstruction* due to formation of a haematoma which compresses the trachea (bleeding is usually from a branch of the superior thyroid artery). Pressure on the trachea can be relieved by removing the skin clips or sutures and evacuating the haematoma. It may be necessary to do this immediately without waiting for a surgeon. If this is unsuccessful, endotracheal intubation is required; however, this may be difficult if the trachea is displaced, and a tracheostomy may have to be performed.

2. *Damage to recurrent laryngeal nerves.* This should be suspected if the vocal cords were not seen to move at extubation. It may be noted early in recovery by asking the patient to answer questions; if the recurrent laryngeal nerves are

damaged, hoarseness or whispering will be evident. In more severe cases there may be stridor, and if both nerves are damaged bilateral abductor paralysis can cause obstruction of the airway, in which case re-intubation will be required. Damage to the cords is more likely following surgery for malignancy or in repeat operations.

3. *Collapsed trachea (tracheomalacia)*. This may only become evident following extubation and may first be noticed in the recovery room. It is a rare complication and tends to occur when a very large thyroid has been removed. Re-intubation will be required until more definitive management can be arranged.

Thyroid Crisis or Storm

Thyroid crisis or storm is rarely seen when the patient is adequately treated with anithyroid drugs pre-operatively and made euthyroid. The presenting features include tachycardia, hypertension, pyrexia, dyspnoea, confusion, dilated pupils and agitation. Management should be started without delay and should include:

1. Intravenous fluid replacement
2. Oxygen therapy and possibly artificial ventilation
3. Potassium iodide
4. α- and β-blockade
5. Cooling by tepid sponging and fanning
6. Hydrocortisone
7. Sodium bicarbonate to correct metabolic acidosis
8. Sedation

Once the condition has been stabilised, the patient's transfer to an intensive care unit will be required for further management.

Dental and Faciomaxillary Surgery

Post-operative Bleeding

Because continued bleeding within the mouth is common, it is particularly important that these patients are nursed on the side with a slight head-down tilt until they regain consciousness so that blood does not pool in the pharynx.

A dental mouth pack may be in place at the end of surgery. This must not be allowed to obstruct the airway. Complete respiratory obstruction has been recorded when, unknown to the recovery staff, a pharyngeal pack has been inadvertently left in place following extubation.

Persistent bleeding may require further surgical intervention. It is particularly dangerous if the blood is being swallowed as this may go unnoticed (see

'Tonsillectomy', p. 118). Gentle suction with a soft suction catheter may be required. This can be conveniently applied via a nasopharyngeal airway or via a shortened nasotracheal tube pulled back so that its tip lies in the pharynx and with a safety pin through it at the nares.

Wiring of the Jaw

Following the reduction of mandibular fractures, facial bone reconstructions and mandibular osteotomies, stabilising wires (usually two or more on either side) are inserted to hold the jaw in a fixed position. Recovery staff should know the position of these wires as they may have to cut them if respiratory obstruction or vomiting occurs. Wire cutters should accompany the patient from the operating theatre and be readily available.

A tongue switch may also be inserted to allow the tongue to be pulled forwards should it obstruct the airway.

Vomiting is particularly hazardous when the jaws are wired, and the prophylactic use of anti-emetics can be useful. Suction can be applied via a nasopharyngeal airway.

Fracture of Zygomatic Arch

Following reduction of the fracture the patient is nursed with the affected side uppermost to avoid pressure on the fracture side.

Mentally Handicapped Patients

Mentally handicapped patients, both adults and children, who require dental treatment under general anaesthesia, need great care during the recovery period. The early administration of analgesics is helpful. As a significant number of these patients will be carriers of Hepatitis B antigen, appropriate precautions should be taken to avoid contamination with their blood or saliva.

Ophthalmic Surgery

Although some ophthalmic surgery is carried out under local anaesthesia, an increasing number of patients receive general anaesthesia. They embrace the extremes of age and include a high proportion of diabetics. As their sight is impaired, frequent explanations and quiet reassurance from the nursing staff will aid smooth recovery.

Position. Until they are fully conscious, patients should be nursed in the lateral position on the unaffected side. This will reduce the likelihood of direct pressure being applied to the eye and should vomiting occur, the operated eye will not be contaminated.

Intra-ocular pressure (IOP). Vomiting, coughing and straining can all cause an unwanted rise in IOP. The pharynx is thoroughly suctioned prior to extubation to minimise pharyngeal stimulation during recovery. Anti-emetic and anti-tussive agents can be employed prophylactically to reduce the incidence of vomiting and coughing.

Pupil size. This may be affected by eye drops given before or during surgery, including:

1. Mydriatics e.g. cyclopentolate and phenylephrine used to dilate pupils for retinal detachment surgery
2. Miotics, e.g. pilocarpine used to constrict pupils in glaucoma

Analgesia. Pain is seldom severe after ophthalmic surgery except following correction of squint and retinal detachment. Children should be restrained from removing dressings and their co-operation sought by gentle persuasion.

Drug interactions. Staff should be aware of drugs used in ophthalmology which may influence the patient's recovery. These include:

1. Ecothiopate, an anticholinesterase used in the treatment of glaucoma which will cause prolonged neuromuscular block if suxamethonium (succinylcholine) has been used.
2. Timolol, a β-blocking drug used in the treatment of glaucoma, can cause bradycardia.

Neurosurgery

Following neurosurgery, changes in intracranial pressure may occur which may be life-threatening if they go undetected. In specialised neurosurgical units, direct intracranial pressure monitoring may be employed. Elsewhere, reliance must be placed in frequent clinical observations which may reflect intracranial events.

For this reason, patients who have undergone craniotomy or who have received a head injury require more detailed post-operative monitoring than others. In addition to the standard observations of pulse, blood pressure and respiratory rate, regular examinations of the pupils and level of consciousness must be continued even after the effects of anaesthesia have apparently worn off. A neurological observation chart based on the Glasgow Coma Scale (see Fig. 5.3) provides a convenient way of recording these observations.

The following signs reflect intracranial events which may require intervention and should be brought to the attention of the neurosurgeon:

1. Deterioration in the level of consciousness
2. Lateralising signs, especially pupillary dilatation
3. Rising blood pressure accompanied by falling pulse rate (Cushing's ischaemic reflex)

4. Changes in the respiratory pattern such as irregular breathing or a slowing of the respiratory rate

It may become necessary to reduce intracranial pressure during the recovery period. The following methods are available:

1. Intravenous mannitol 0.25–0.5 g/kg over 30 min
2. Intravenous dexamethasone 10 mg
3. Intravenous frusemide (furosemide) 20–40 mg
4. Intubation followed by controlled hyperventilation to maintain $PaCO_2$ at between 3.3 and 4 kPa. A neurological assessment should be made before sedatives or muscle relaxants are given since these drugs mask the signs of rising intracranial pressure

Recovery staff must be alert for any factors which may cause an undesirable rise in intracranial pressure in the post-operative period. These include:

1. Hypoxia and hypercarbia due to respiratory obstruction or ventilatory impairment
2. Increased venous pressure due to coughing or straining, the head-down position or circulatory overload
3. Hypertension or hypotension sufficient to interfere with autoregulation or cerebral blood supply

Care in the post-operative period should therefore be directed towards:

1. *Ensuring adequate respiration*
   a) Careful attention to maintenance of a clear airway
   b) Administration of oxygen
   c) Blood gas analysis. If hypoxia or hypercarbia occur, controlled ventilation may be required

2. *Avoidance of increased venous pressure*
   a) Patients should be nursed in a slight head-up position to encourage venous drainage
   b) Cautious intravenous fluid administration to avoid circulatory overload
   c) Prevention of coughing and straining. If an oropharyngeal airway or endotracheal tube causes irritation it should be taken out or the patient adequately sedated. Secretions must be promptly removed by suction catheter.

3. *Avoidance of excessive hypertension.* Hypotensive agents must be used with extreme caution following neurosurgery. Hypertension may be a sign of Cushing's ischaemic reflex and reducing the blood pressure may further prejudice brain stem perfusion; consequently, investigation, e.g. brain scan or angiography, should precede treatment. Hypertension is frequently seen after aneurysm surgery with induced hypotension. Injudicious hypotensive therapy may cause vasospasm of the feeding vessels when the blood pressure falls, with resulting hemiparesis.

   In extreme cases, where hypotensive therapy is unavoidable, the patient should be transferred to an intensive therapy unit since continuous blood pressure monitoring is essential.

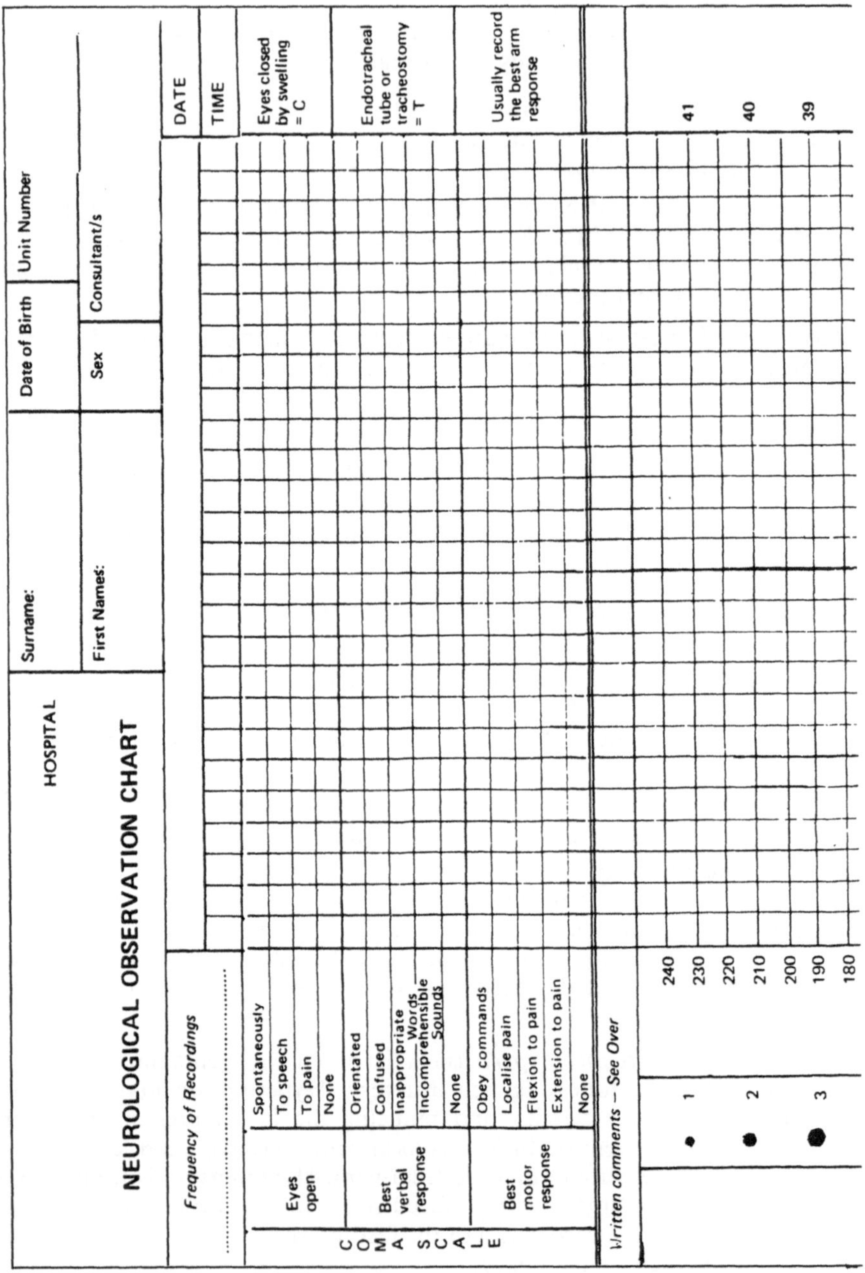

Fig. 5.3. Neurological observation chart.

NEUROLOGICAL OBSERVATION CHART

HOSPITAL

Surname:

First Names:

Date of Birth | Unit Number

Sex | Consultant/s

DATE

TIME

Frequency of Recordings

Eyes open	Spontaneously	
	To speech	
	To pain	
	None	
Best verbal response	Orientated	
	Confused	
	Inappropriate Words	
	Incomprehensible Sounds	
	None	
Best motor response	Obey commands	
	Localise pain	
	Flexion to pain	
	Extension to pain	
	None	

C
O
M
A

S
C
A
L
E

Eyes closed by swelling = C

Endotracheal tube or tracheostomy = T

Usually record the best arm response

41
40
39

240
230
220
210
200
190
180

Written comments — See Over

1
2
3

Temperature °C: 38, 37, 36, 35, 34, 33, 32, 31

+ reacts
− no reaction
c. eye closed by swelling

Record right (R) and left (L) separately if there is a difference between the two sides.

Blood pressure and Pulse rate: 170, 160, 150, 140, 130, 120, 110, 100, 90, 80, 70, 60, 50, 40, 30

Respiration 20, 10

Pupil Scale (m.m.): 4, 5, 6, 7, 8

PUPILS		
right	Size	
	Reaction	
left	Size	
	Reaction	

LIMB MOVEMENT		
ARMS	Normal power	
	Mild weakness	
	Severe weakness	
	Spastic flexion	
	Extension	
	No response	
LEGS	Normal power	
	Mild weakness	
	Severe weakness	
	Extension	
	No response	

Temperature changes. Recovery from neurosurgery may be characterised by disturbed body temperature regulation. Constant monitoring and correction, if necessary, are required.

Hyperthermia may follow surgery in the region of the temperature-regulating centre in the hypothalamus, whereas hypothermia may result from long anaesthesia and active cooling. Shivering should be avoided since this causes an increase in oxygen requirements. Sedation and controlled ventilation may be necessary to prevent this.

Convulsions may result from cerebral damage or oedema and should be managed in the standard way (see p. 97).

Thoracic Surgery

Bronchoscopy

The anaesthetic technique should provide a rapid return of the cough reflex post-operatively. If, however, topical or local anaesthesia has been used, the full return of reflexes may take several hours. The patient should be nursed in the lateral head-down position.

Post-operative complications include:

1. Laryngospasm (see p. 68)
2. Laryngeal oedema, especially in children (see pp. 68 and 135)
3. Bleeding. If this is severe the surgeon and the anaesthetist must be informed. Treatment may include the introduction of an endobronchial blocker into the affected lung and ventilation of the other lung via an endotracheal tube
4. Perforation of the bronchus. The presenting features may include dyspnoea, retrosternal pain or surgical emphysema. The surgeon should be informed if perforation of the bronchus is suspected.

Thoracotomy

Chest Drains

Following thoracic surgery, chest drains are usually inserted to enable air and fluid, including blood, to escape from the pleural cavity. They are normally positioned as follows:

1. Apical or upper drain to facilitate drainage of air
2. Posterior or lower drain to facilitate drainage of blood

A number of drainage systems are in use:

1. The simple underwater seal drainage bottle (Fig. 5.4)
2. The Heimlich flutter valve – a disposable valve which allows air or blood to escape outwards but prevents air re-entering the pleural cavity
3. The Pleurevac system – a sterile disposable plastic unit

Drainage through an underwater seal can be aided by attaching a mechanical pump (e.g. the Roberts pump) to the open end to provide continuous suction. The use of a suction pump is not advised following pneumonectomy as it may lead to gross mediastinal shift.

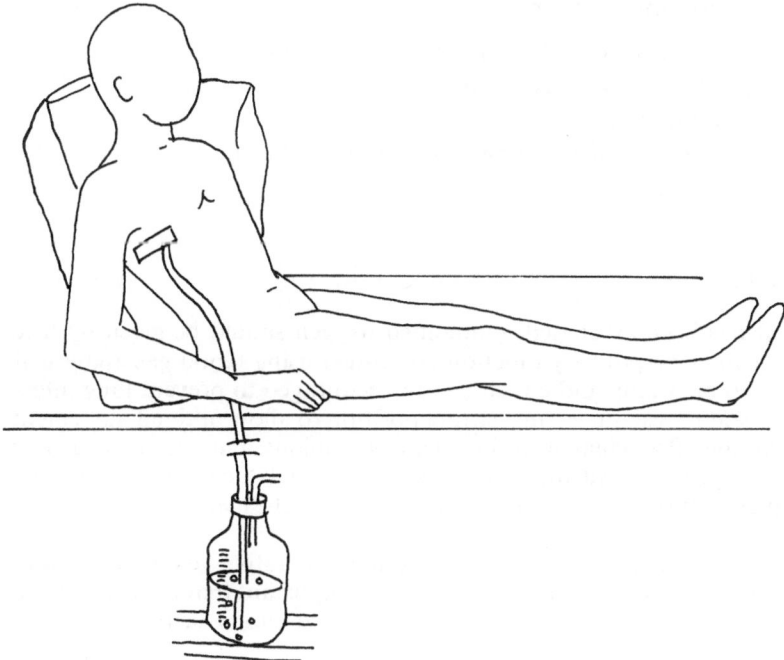

Fig. 5.4. Underwater seal drain.

If the drainage tube is patent, the meniscus in the tube should rise and fall in time with respiration and this should be checked regularly. If the tube becomes blocked, it may be cleared by 'milking' it with roller clamps, in the direction away from the patient.

Fluid from the drainage bottle must not be allowed to re-enter the pleural cavity; this can be ensured by keeping the bottle on the floor beneath the patient's bed. The tubing must be double clamped when the patient is being moved.

The volume of fluid escaping is measured using graduations on the side of the bottle. Changes in the fluid level should be recorded. There should be intermittent bubbling of air through the underwater seal, in time with respiration. Continuous bubbling throughout the respiratory cycle in a ventilated patient is indicative of a bronchopleural leak and the tidal volume may need to be increased.

The patient should be nursed in the supine position with gradual elevation to 45° as normal reflexes and consciousness return. This will aid lung expansion and facilitate fluid drainage.

X-ray

When the initial assessment of the patient has been completed, an X-ray of the chest should be taken in order to:

1. Confirm that re-expansion of the lungs has occurred
2. Check the position of the mediastinum
3. Exclude pneumothorax
4. Ascertain the position of the chest drains and CVP catheter
5. Reveal hidden bleeding

Respiratory System

If the patient has been extubated, humidified oxygen should be given by face mask and adequate respiratory function confirmed using blood gas analysis if necessary. Deep breathing and coughing are encouraged to prevent lung infections. The patient is best nursed in a sitting position to allow optimal movement of the diaphragm. Bronchial secretions can be copious and the trachea may need frequent aspiration. Adequate analgesia is essential and epidural narcotics or the intrapleural infusion of local anaesthetic may be the methods of choice (p. 62).

If the patient requires a period of elective post-operative ventilation, endotracheal suction should take place regularly. It is important that the catheter tip passes beyond the end of the endotracheal tube and enters each bronchus in turn.

Cardiovascular System

Blood loss may be extensive during thoracotomy and may continue post-operatively. Blood transfusion should be given as indicated by the clinical findings and not simply by the amount of blood lost in the chest drains.

Hypothermia

Heat loss during surgery may be considerable and hypothermia is managed as previously described (p. 98).

Pain Relief

The importance of adequate pain relief after thoracic surgery cannot be over emphasised. Such surgery is potentially extremely painful and if analgesia is inadequate the patient will not breathe sufficiently, cough or co-operate with the physiotherapist. The patient should be alert and pain-free when he leaves the recovery unit and, thereafter, analgesia should be matched to his individual requirements.

Vascular Surgery

The post-operative recovery of patients who have undergone the surgical repair of an aortic aneurysm is described, although the same general principles apply to other forms of vascular surgery.

Patients requiring aortic surgery are usually elderly with generalised arterial disease so that a history of hypertension and myocardial ischaemia is common. Post-operatively they are frequently transferred directly to an intensive care unit where elective ventilation may be continued until cardiovascular stability returns. If, however, intensive care facilities are not available, patients must be monitored closely in the recovery room until they are ready to return to the ward.

Oxygen therapy is given routinely and respiratory performance monitored by blood gas analysis. Arterial blood samples should not, however, be taken from the femoral artery as grafts may be damaged.

The following problems may be encountered:

1. *Hypertension* is frequently seen post-operatively, possibly owing to renin release after aortic cross-clamping. It will put an unnecessary strain on the graft and is particularly dangerous in patients with myocardial ischaemia. Active measures are taken to reduce the blood pressure to normal values (see p. 82).

2. *Hypotension* is commonly due to inadequate blood replacement. Bleeding may continue post-operatively; the drainage bottles must be carefully watched and blood loss measured and replaced. It must be remembered that concealed bleeding may be significant. The pulse rate and central venous pressure measurements provide a useful guide to replacement.

3. *Oliguria*. Renal perfusion may have been impaired by cross-clamping of the aorta or by hypovolaemia. Urine output is monitored and maintained above a minimum of 0.5 ml/(kg·h) (see p. 108). A 'renal' dose of dopamine (2–3 μg/(kg·min)) is often given prophylactically.

4. *Hypothermia* may be due to long bowel exposure and large transfusions of cold blood and will result in vasoconstriction with further hypertension, myocardial depression and irritability (see p. 98).

5. *Failure of coagulation*. Following intra-operative heparinisation and the transfusion of large volumes of blood, coagulation may be impaired post-

operatively. If persistent bleeding is a problem, blood samples are taken for coagulation studies and the appropriate replacement therapy given (see p. 104).

6. *Electrolyte imbalance* may be due to massive blood transfusion, diuretic therapy or hypothermia. Blood is taken in the early post-operative period for electrolyte estimation so that abnormalities can be detected and corrections made where necessary.

7. *Metabolic acidosis* due to impaired circulation in the lower limbs when the aorta is cross-clamped. This may result in impaired myocardial contraction and difficulty in reversing non-depolarising muscle relaxants. Sodium bicarbonate is used to correct severe degrees of metabolic acidosis using the formula $1/3 \times$ body weight (kg) $\times$ base deficit $=$ mmol of sodium bicarbonate required. This is usually given in small increments, and progress is monitored by serial measurements to prevent overcorrection.

8. *Thrombus formation.* The limbs must be frequently inspected for signs of impaired circulation (pallor, cyanosis, drop in temperature), and the pulses felt (see p. 25). A Doppler ultrasonic device may prove useful in detecting thrombus formation. The surgeon must be informed if the peripheral circulation appears impaired as further surgery may be indicated.

Pain Relief

Continuous analgesia via an epidural catheter is frequently used following aortic surgery. The catheter must be positioned pre-operatively before the patient is heparinised to avoid the possibility of neurological damage due to haematoma formation. This method of pain relief has the additional advantage of improving blood flow due to sympathetic blockade but recovery staff must be aware of the further implications (see p. 60).

Intramuscular opiates will be poorly absorbed if tissue perfusion is impaired post-operatively; small increments given intravenously will be more effective.

Genito-urinary Surgery

Prostatectomy

Most prostatic surgery is performed via the transurethral route using a resectoscope. As many patients who require this type of surgery are old and may have significant respiratory or cardiac disease, epidural or spinal anaesthesia is frequently employed.

Bladder irrigation. In order to prevent clots of blood blocking the urinary catheter following prostatectomy, the bladder is continuously irrigated. Warming the irrigation fluid will minimise heat loss and vasoconstriction. The volume of irrigation fluid instilled into the bladder and the volume drained must be recorded and any discrepancy noted. Such discrepancies may occur if the bladder has been perforated.

Bladder distension may cause patients to feel they need to micturate. They may worry they will become incontinent and constant reassurance is required.

The abdomen should be inspected periodically for signs of excessive bladder distension. Manual compression of the bladder may aid drainage, especially following spinal or epidural anaesthesia. If the catheter becomes blocked by clots, these should be removed without delay using a bladder syringe. If this is difficult or incomplete, the patient must return to the theatre for operative removal of the clots.

Fluid balance. Large volumes of fluid may be absorbed from the prostatic bed during and after surgery with the danger of circulatory overload. As the absorbed fluid may contain little sodium, a dilutional hyponatraemia can result. This is characterised by restlessness and confusion, leading to convulsions and coma. Treatment is with hypertonic saline (sodium chloride 1.8%) and diuretics.

Blood pressure. Hypotensive anaesthesia is frequently employed to reduce bleeding during prostatectomy. The blood pressure should be allowed to rise slowly during the post-operative period as a sudden rise in pressure may provoke brisk haemorrhage and increase the chances of clot formation. As blood loss may continue during the recovery period, the circulating volume must be maintained with intravenous fluids (p. 42). Sodium chloride 0.9% is suitable as it helps maintain sodium levels. If bleeding is excessive, blood transfusion will be required. Traction on the catheter will exert pressure on the prostatic bed and aid the control of bleeding. The surgeon should be kept informed of persistent bleeding as further surgery may be indicated.

Perforated bladder. This may follow prostate or bladder surgery and must be suspected if the following occur:

1. Increasing pulse rate
2. Hypotension
3. Abdominal pain and tenderness. This may be masked following spinal or epidural anaesthesia. There may be upper abdominal or shoulder pain due to irritation of the diaphragm with irrigation fluids.
4. Abdominal distension with absent bowel sounds
5. Continuous small deficits in bladder irrigation fluid measurements. The irrigation should be stopped and the surgeon informed without delay.

Disseminated intravascular coagulation (DIC) or fibrinolysis may follow prostatectomy owing to the absorption of prostatic tissue into the circulation. DIC will cause persistent bleeding and is diagnosed on the basis of the results of a clotting screen (p. 104). The prostatic bed is sometimes perfused with a solution containing aminocaproic acid to prevent this complication.

Septic shock. The absorption of endotoxins or bacteria into the circulation at prostatectomy may lead to septic shock, which is characterised by pyrexia, tachycardia, hypotension and a weak thready pulse. Vigorous antibiotic therapy and intravenous fluid therapy will be required. If there is no improvement despite adequate hydration and the CVP is high, inotropic support with a dopamine infusion may be helpful. Urine output should be maintained above 0.5 ml/(kg·h) using diuretics if necessary. Following initial resuscitation, transfer to an intensive care unit is recommended.

Nephrectomy

Atelectasis of the lower lung may occur when this operation is performed with the patient on one side in the jack-knife position. Early post-operative physiotherapy with adequate analgesia will help re-expand the lung.

A post-operative chest X-ray is taken to exclude pneumothorax resulting from accidental damage to the pleura. Should a pneumothorax be found, it will be necessary to insert a chest drain with an underwater seal.

Circumcision

It is both easy and satisfying to provide excellent post-operative analgesia for children who undergo circumcision. Penile blocks and caudal epidural analgesia are equally safe and effective (pp. 61 and 62).

Paediatric Surgery

Post-operatively in paediatric patients, special attention must be paid, not only to maintaining adequate respiratory and cardiovascular function, but also to temperature regulation and fluid balance.

Maintenance of Airway and Adequacy of Ventilation

When assessing respiratory function in infants as opposed to adults it should be remembered that:

1. The ribs are horizontal and breathing is mainly diaphragmatic
2. Respiratory rates between 30 and 40 per minute are normal
3. The narrowest point of the upper airway is at the cricoid cartilage

Face masks and nasal cannulae are unsatisfactory in conscious patients and if oxygen therapy is required an incubator, tent or face tent should be used. An incubator is preferable for smaller infants as temperature, oxygen therapy and humidity are more easily controlled, but a tent is needed for larger infants.

The following may be required for airway management and should be readily available:

Table 5.1. Endotracheal tube sizes

Age (years)	Internal diameter of tube (mm)
Neonate	3.0
1	4.0
2	5.0
4	5.5
6	6.0
8	6.5
10	7.0
12	7.5

Tube length oral $= 12 + \dfrac{age}{2}$ cm

nasal $= 13.5 + \dfrac{age}{2}$ cm

1. Range of paediatric oral airways
2. Range of anaesthetic face masks
3. Range of endotracheal tubes and introducers (Table 5.1). It may be wise for the paediatric anaesthetic circuit, laryngoscope, endotracheal tube and mask to accompany the patient from the operating theatre to the recovery unit.
4. Paediatric laryngoscope
5. Paediatric anaesthetic circuit or Ambu bag so that assisted ventilation can be given either by face mask or via endotracheal tube
6. Fine suction catheters that can pass through endotracheal tubes

The causes of respiratory inadequacy found in paediatric patients are essentially the same as those found in adults (see p. 67). Similarly, management is directed towards:

1. *Ensuring a clear airway* by inserting an oropharyngeal airway, supporting the jaw and removing any foreign matter by suction.
2. *Assisting inadequate respiratory efforts* by giving intermittent positive pressure ventilation via a face mask and reservoir bag. This should take precedence over attempts at intubation, which is seldom necessary and should only be attempted by those with adequate experience.

Post-extubation sub-glottic or laryngeal oedema. The incidence of this serious complication has been reduced by the use of endotracheal tubes made of non-irritant material, e.g. PVC, and of a size that allows a slight air leak. Oedema is more likely if there have been difficulties with intubation or if there is an upper respiratory tract infection; it must be recognised and treated promptly because of the danger of respiratory obstruction.

The first signs frequently appear within 2 h of extubation and include:

1. Inspiratory stridor
2. Croupy cough

3. Rib retraction
4. Restlessness
5. Pallor or cyanosis

Treatment includes:

1. Oxygen
2. Humidity
3. Head-up position to increase venous drainage
4. Diuretics
5. Dexamethasone
6. Antibiotics
7. Nebulised adrenaline (racemic epinephrine)

The use of sedatives is not recommended. If this treatment is unsuccessful, intubation is required to bypass the obstruction.

Loose teeth present a frequent hazard and are best removed in a controlled way while the child is still unconscious in case they fall out during recovery and are inhaled. Teeth should be saved and returned to the ward with the patient for the attention of the Tooth Fairy.

Maintenance of Adequate Cardiovascular Function

Although the same general principles of assessing cardiovascular function in adults (p. 24) apply in paediatric patients, certain differences should be borne in mind:

1. The normal heart rate is faster (Table 5.2). This can conveniently be monitored using a precordial stethoscope which will, in addition, allow breath sounds to be heard.

Table 5.2. Relationship of heart rate to age

Age	Approximate heart rate
Birth	140 per minute
One month	130 per minute
1 year	120 per minute
2 years	110 per minute
4 years	100 per minute
8 years	90 per minute
12 years	80 per minute

2. The blood pressure is lower (Table 5.3). When measuring the blood pressure it is essential that the correct size of cuff is used (see Table 2. 3). The blood pressure can be measured using a stethoscope on the brachial artery or with a suitable automatic device e.g. Dinamap.

Table 5.3. Relationship of blood pressure to age

Age	Approx. blood pressure (mmHg)
Birth	75/45
one month	80/50
1 year	85/60
2 years	90/60
4 years	95/60
8 years	100/60
12 years	110/65

3. The margin of safety following haemorrhage is less. Because of the small total blood volume, a comparatively small blood loss in absolute terms can represent a considerable proportion of the total circulating blood volume. Measuring blood loss must be precise and early fluid replacement will be required to prevent hypovolaemia.

4. The heart is especially sensitive to vagally-mediated bradycardia following upper airway stimulation and suxamethonium (succinylcholine). The heart rate usually recovers quickly but atropine may be required and should be readily available. Continuous ECG monitoring will give an early warning of changes of heart rate or rhythm but it must be remembered that it indicates electrical activity and gives no indication of the mechanical efficiency of the heart.

Temperature Regulation

Small children have a greater tendency than adults to lose heat during surgery because:

1. They have a proportionally greater surface area to mass
2. Their temperature-regulating centre is underdeveloped
3. They have less subcutaneous fatty tissue
4. Their ability to shiver and so regenerate heat is less well developed

They are frequently cold when they arrive in the recovery room so it is particularly important that their temperature is monitored post-operatively. Low temperatures must be corrected before the patient is allowed to return to the ward (p. 98).

Conversely, high temperatures may be found in children and these must also be detected and treated, as cerebral hypoxia or convulsions may follow (see p. 99). A raised temperature may also indicate that the child is developing malignant hyperthermia (p. 100).

Fluid Balance

In addition to the replacement of blood and fluids lost before and during surgery, the basic fluid maintenance requirements should be given to all children except those undergoing very minor surgery who may be expected to drink again soon after they recover from their anaesthetic.

Normal maintenance values (Table 5.4) can be used as a guideline but must be adjusted according to individual circumstances, e.g. dehydration and pyrexia. Hartmann's solution or 0.9% sodium chloride should not normally be given but dextrose/saline solutions (0.18% or 0.45% NaCl in 5% dextrose) used instead. If there has been a long period of starvation in the peri-operative period, hypoglycaemia may occur. This can be confirmed by using dextrostix and treated with intravenous glucose.

Table 5.4. Maintenance intravenous fluid requirements

1st month of life	6 ml/(kg·h) (during the first week the requirements are less. Multiply age in days)
	$\dfrac{}{7}$
After the first month	
< 10 kg	4 ml/(kg·h)
10–20 kg	3 ml/(kg·h)
20–30 kg	2 ml/(kg·h)
> 30 kg	1.5 ml/(kg·h)

A reliable infusion site is essential and the cannula should be secured by adequate strapping and splinting in such a way that inspection of the puncture site and the rapid detection of the extravasation of infused solutions are possible. A butterfly needle is easily displaced and is not recommended for a prolonged infusion.

Some method of volume limitation should be used to prevent accidental overloading of the circulation, especially in infants and small children. The Metriset allows a convenient method of administration of small volumes of fluid and provides a degree of safety as the chamber will require refilling periodically, but for greater reliability an infusion pump such as the IVAC is recommended.

Further Reading

Atkinson RS (1979) Post-operative care. In: Hewer CL, Atkinson RS (eds) Recent advances in anaesthesia and analgesia, no. 13. Churchill Livingstone, Edinburgh, pp 185–197
Atkinson RS, Rushman GB, Lee J Alfred (1982) A synopsis of anaesthesia, 9th edn. Wright, Bristol
Brown TCK, Fisk GC (1979) Anaesthesia for children, including aspects of intensive care. Blackwell Scientific, Oxford, pp 135–140
Churchill-Davidson HC (ed) (1978) A practice of anaesthesia, 4th edn. Lloyd-Luke, London
Enderby GEH (1985) Hypotensive anaesthesia. Churchill Livingstone, London
Gothard JWW, Branthwaite MA (1982) Anaesthesia for thoracic surgery. Blackwell Scientific Publications, London
Hatch DJ (1981) Anaesthetic equipment for neonates and infants. Br J Hosp Med 26: 84–88
Jewkes D (1987) Anaesthesia for neurosurgery. Clinical Anaesthesiology. Bailliere Tindall, New York

Miller RD (1981) Anaesthesia. Churchill Livingstone, New York

Morrison JD, Mirakur RK, Craig HJL (1985) Anaesthesia for eye, ear, nose and throat surgery. Churchill Livingstone, London

Rees G Jackson, Gray TC (1981) Paediatric anaesthesia: Trends in current practice. Butterworths, London

Selwyn Crawford J (1984) Obstetric analgesia and anaesthesia. Churchill Livingstone, London

Smith GB (1983) Ophthalmic anaesthesia. Arnold, London

Steward DJ (1979) Manual of paediatric anaesthesia. Churchill Livingstone, New York, Edinburgh, London

Walters FJM, Nott MR (1977) The hazards of anesthesia in the injured patient. Br J Anaesth 49: 707–720

Willatts SM, Walters FJM (1986) Anaesthesia and intensive care for the neurosurgical patient. Blackwell Scientific Publications, London

Chapter 6

Pre-existing Factors Affecting Recovery

Premedication

The type and dosage of drugs given as premedication can influence recovery from anaesthesia in many ways:

1. *A relative overdose of depressant drugs* relative to the patient's age and weight is one of many causes of a delayed return of consciousness (p. 93). This is particularly true when large doses of narcotic analgesic agents are given to the frail and elderly, but relative overdose may also follow benzodiazepine, phenothiazine or hyoscine (scopolamine) administration. Reversal of the effects of opiates can be achieved by intravenous naloxone (0.1–0.4 mg) or doxapram (50–100 mg).

Benzodiazepines can be reversed by the recently introduced specific antagonist flumazenil. Like naloxone, it should be administered slowly until the desired effect is obtained. The usual dose is 300–600 µg.

2. *Long-acting premedicating agents* whose action may persist into the postoperative period, especially if the surgical procedure is brief. Examples include droperidol and lorazepam.

3. *Anti-sialogogues*. When anti-sialogogues have been omitted, recovery may be accompanied by excessive salivation, especially following intubation, oral surgery and certain premedications e.g. lorazepam. Frequent suction may be necessary to maintain a clear airway and to prevent coughing and laryngeal irritation.

Anaesthetic Technique

Intravenous Induction Agents

When propofol has been used for induction of anaesthesia, recovery is generally rapid as the agent is quickly metabolised. This is obviously an advantage especially in patients who are having day surgery. However, if analgesics have not been given intra-operatively, they may be needed as soon as the patient awakes.

Long-acting Inhalational Agents

The higher the blood : gas solubility ratio of inhalational agents, the slower is their rate of elimination. Return of consciousness will therefore be prolonged following the use of the more soluble agents such as trichlorethylene and diethyl ether. Less soluble agents such as halothane, enflurane and isoflurane allow a more rapid recovery.

Analgesic and Relaxant Technique

A much lighter plane of anaesthesia can be achieved with a nitrous oxide-relaxant-hyperventilation technique with opiate supplements than by allowing a patient to breathe volatile agents spontaneously. Recovery of consciousness is correspondingly quicker.

Regional Anaesthesia

Patients who have been rendered pain-free by regional techniques, e.g. caudal anaesthesia, will tend to sleep peacefully once consciousness has returned, free of the restlessness and hypertension which characterise the patient in pain. This is especially valuable in children following painful operations such as circumcision. When spinal or epidural anaesthesia have been used, in addition to the sensory block, a degree of motor and autonomic block may persist into the post-operative period. It is important for recovery staff to be aware of this because:

1. The patient may be alarmed at his inability to move and will require reassurance.
2. Sudden changes in posture may cause hypotension.
3. Hypovolaemia must not be allowed to occur as compensatory vasoconstriction is impaired.
4. Urinary retention is common.

Brachial plexus block may persist well after completion of surgery and the arm may need to be supported in a sling for protection until motor function has returned. If the supraclavicular approach has been used, pneumothorax is a potential side-effect that may not become obvious until the patient is in the recovery room. Such patients may also notice voice changes due to recurrent laryngeal nerve blockade.

Induced Hypotension

Deliberate hypotension used to facilitate surgery and reduce blood loss can be achieved in many ways including:

1. *Depression of myocardial contractility* (negative inotropic effect), e.g. by halothane, β-blocking agents
2. *Sympathetic blockade* by ganglion-blocking agents, e.g. trimetaphan or by spinal or epidural anaesthesia
3. *Vasodilating drugs*, e.g. isoflurane, α-blocking agents, nitroprusside, nitro-glycerine

Following the use of these techniques, patients may arrive in the recovery unit with some degree of residual hypotension. Providing there is no hypovolaemia and peripheral perfusion is good, the blood pressure can normally be allowed to rise slowly as the agents are eliminated. A sudden rise in blood pressure may provoke unwanted haemorrhage. These patients do not tolerate sudden changes in posture and, in particular, they should not sit up until the effects of the hypotensive agents have worn off. It should be remembered that patients who have received ganglion-blocking agents may have widely dilated pupils un-responsive to light.

If persistent or excessive hypotension occurs:

1. Give oxygen by face mask
2. Elevate foot of bed to improve venous return
3. Increase rate of intravenous fluid administration

Subsequent treatment will depend on the mechanism of action of the drugs used and may consist of:

1. Positive inotropic agents, e.g. 10% calcium gluconate up to 10 ml slowly i.v.
2. Direct-acting vasoconstrictors, e.g. methoxamine 20 mg diluted in 500ml sodium chloride 0.9%
3. Drugs combining both actions, e.g. ephedrine in increments of 5–10 mg i.v.

Ketamine

Patients who have been given ketamine may remain unconscious for several hours. To reduce emergence delirium, which is exacerbated by unwarranted stimulation, they should be nursed in a quiet corner of the recovery room until consciousness has returned. Disturbing hallucinations can be minimised by intravenous diazepam (see p. 3).

Pre-operative Drug Therapy

Anti-hypertensive Agents

Drugs used to lower blood pressure may act either by reducing the tone in the peripheral vessels, e.g. guanethidine, methyldopa and ACE inhibitors, or by reducing the force of cardiac contraction, e.g. β-blockers.

1. *Drugs reducing peripheral vascular tone.* The ability of vessels to constrict in response to hypovolaemia or hypotension is impaired. Blood volume must be maintained post-operatively. Severe hypotension in the absence of hypo-volaemia can be treated with direct-acting vasoconstricting agents such as methoxamine.

2. *β-blocking agents.* If severe bradycardia or hypotension occurs in patients on β-blockers, additional β-stimulation can be provided by an isoprenaline (isoproterenol) infusion under ECG monitoring. Circulating volume must be maintained.

Monoamine Oxidase Inhibitors (MAOIs)

Examples of MAOIs include pargyline, phenelzine and tranylcypromine.

Extreme care should be taken if using pethidine (meperidine) and morphine derivatives for post-operative analgesia in patients receiving MAOI therapy. Many reactions to such combinations have been reported, including:

1. Muscle twitching
2. Hypotension
3. Ataxia
4. Cerebral excitation
5. Coma
6. Respiratory depression

If no alternative method of post-operative analgesia is effective, a small test dose of pethidine, e.g. 5 mg, may be tried. if there is no abnormal reaction further increments may be given at 5-min intervals until sufficient analgesia is produced.

Patients taking MAOIs may also develop marked hypertension if given pressor agents and care is thus recommended with:

1. Ephedrine
2. Amphetamines
3. L-dopa

Adrenaline (epinephrine), however, is not harmful as it is metabolised by catechol-*O*-methyltransferase to monoamine oxidase.

Corticosteroids

The amount of hydrocortisone secreted in response to surgery may be as high as 400 mg/day. Patients on long-term steroid therapy and those who have received a course of steroids within the previous 6 months can develop adrenocortical insufficiency in the immediate post-operative period. Such patients may be unable to respond to the stress of anaesthesia and surgery and will require supplemental steroids.

Steroid cover in the form of hydrocortisone hemisuccinate 100 mg i.m. can be given with the premedication and repeated 6-hourly for 2 days following major surgery and for 24 hours following minor surgery. For a very brief procedure a single injection should be sufficient.

The blood pressure should be carefully monitored following surgery in this group of patients since adrenocortical insufficiency may present as hypotension unexplained by other causes. Treatment is by a bolus of hydrocortisone 100–200 mg and intravenous fluids.

Insulin and Hypoglycaemic Agents

See Diabetes Mellitus, p. 152

Anticoagulants

1. *Heparin*. This is used as prophylaxis against deep vein thrombosis and pulmonary embolism (see p. 82). A dose of 5000 units subcutaneously before surgery should not cause bleeding problems post-operatively. Full anticoagulation with heparin, as used in cardiovascular surgery, will require reversal with protamine sulphate (p. 104).
2. *Oral anticoagulants* (e.g. warfarin, phenindione). These are used prophylactically in patients with a history of:
   a) Pulmonary embolism
   b) Recurrent thrombophlebitis
   c) Valve disease
   d) Valve replacement

These patients are normally converted to treatment with intravenous heparin before surgery. Oral anticoagulant administration is then ceased. In an emergency, anticoagulation produced by warfarin may be reversed with a transfusion of fresh frozen plasma.

Diuretics

Patients with cardiac failure, ischaemic heart disease and hypertension may be receiving diuretic therapy. If potassium supplementation has been inadequate, hypokalaemia may result in:

1. Cardiac irregularities (p. 89)
2. Prolonged neuromuscular block (p. 72)

In these patients further intravenous potassium replacement will be required.

Antibiotics

Aminoglycoside antibiotics such as gentamicin and neomycin may occasionally prolong the neuromuscular blockade produced by non-depolarising relaxants. Full reversal should always be ensured before patients are allowed to leave the recovery room if they have received these agents. Intravenous calcium may be of value in speeding recovery from neuromuscular block in such patients.

Digoxin

The side-effects of digoxin treatment are greater if the patient is also hypokalaemic. If this occurs in the recovery period, signs of digoxin toxicity (especially dysrhythmias) may occur and urgent intravenous potassium replacement is required.

If inotropic support becomes necessary in a patient already receiving digoxin, further digoxin is inadvisable as toxicity may occur. Dopamine or dobutamine are suitable alternatives.

Respiratory Disease

Chronic Bronchitis

Patients with chronic bronchitis become insensitive to raised $PaCO_2$ levels and rely on a hypoxic drive to stimulate respiration. Uncontrolled oxygen therapy in the recovery period may decrease the normal respiratory drive and lead to hypoventilation. Graded concentrations of oxygen should be administered via a Venturi mask (Fig. 2.12 p. 40) starting with 24%, and progress monitored with a pulse oximeter or by serial blood gas estimations. If respiration is inadequate, doxapram, given either as a bolus or as a continuous infusion, may stimulate respiration but intubation and controlled ventilation may be required until the effects of surgery and anaesthesia have worn off. If opiates are used for post-operative analgesia, extreme caution is needed as respiratory failure may be precipitated. Small intravenous increments should be titrated against the patient's response so avoiding excessive administration. Alternatively, regional anaesthesia may enable adequate pain relief to be achieved without the need for opiates (pp. 61 and 142).

In severe bronchitis a period of elective ventilation in an intensive care unit may be indicated, especially if there is a high abdominal or thoracic incision.

Asthma

Patients suffering from asthma must be particularly closely observed as episodes of bronchospasm may be precipitated by upper airway irritation or drugs (see p. 76). If bronchospasm does occur, high concentrations of oxygen can, and should, be administered.

Cardiovascular Disease

Certain pre-operative factors are now recognised as being associated with an increased risk of ischaemia, infarction or death when patients undergo anaesthesia and surgery. In order of importance these are:

1. A third heart sound or jugular venous distention, i.e. evidence of inadequately treated cardiac failure
2. A myocardial infarction within the preceding six months
3. Rhythms other than sinus or premature atrial contractions
4. More than five ventricular ectopics per minute
5. Age over 70 years
6. Emergency surgery
7. Aortic stenosis
8. Poor general medical condition

Coronary Artery Disease

When myocardial oxygen demand exceeds supply, myocardial ischaemia or infarction will result. Patients with coronary artery disease are particularly prone to develop this complication in the recovery room if:

1. Myocardial oxygen supply is reduced by hypoxaemia or by a diastolic pressure inadequate to perfuse the coronary arteries, or
2. Myocardial oxygen requirements are increased by excessive cardiac workload, e.g. hypertension, tachycardia, shivering

Myocardial ischaemia is best prevented by:

1. Administration of oxygen
2. Maintenance of pulse rate and blood pressure at normal pre-operative values
3. Early and adequate pain relief

Evidence of myocardial ischaemia can be demonstrated by the appearance of depressed ST segments on the ECG.

Hypertension

It is important for the recovery staff to know the pre-operative blood pressure and to relate post-operative measurements to this. Details of anti-hypertensive drug therapy must also be known (see p. 143).

Patients with hypertension have a non-compliant circulation due to atherosclerotic changes in the vessel walls and anti-hypertensive therapy. Changes in circulating volume can result in extreme variations in blood pressure.

The principles of post-operative management include:

1. Frequent blood pressure measurements and prompt correction of any major fluctuations
2. Maintenance of normal circulating volume
3. Adequate analgesia to prevent a hypertensive response to pain

Cardiac Failure

The management of the patient with cardiac failure in the recovery period includes the following:

1. *Administration of oxygen.*
2. *Posture.* A trolley or bed which allows the patient to sit up should be available.
3. *Fluid restriction.* Intravenous fluids must be administered cautiously as circulatory overload can easily be precipitated. Central venous or pulmonary capillary wedge pressure measurements will provide a guide to fluid therapy.
4. *Inotropic support.* When inotropic support is required, digoxin or one of the more rapidly acting agents such as deslanoside can be given intravenously provided the patient is not already digitalised (p. 81). Alternatively dopamine or dobutamine can be used.
5. *Diuretics,* e.g. frusemide (furosemide) 20–40 mg i.v. Catheterisation of the bladder will usually be required.

Pacemaker

Patients who have complete heart block will have a temporary or permanent pacemaker in place. These should present no problems. It is important, however, to prevent any hypovolaemia or postural hypotension as this may lead to a fall in cardiac output if the pacemaker is on a fixed rate.

It is prudent to have available an alternative method of pacing, such as an oesophageal pacing electrode.

Neuromuscular disease

Myasthenia Gravis

Myasthenia gravis is a chronic disease thought to be due to a defect in the synthesis or storage of acetylcholine at the nerve ending. Symptoms include progressive muscular weakness and fatigue. One or more muscle groups may be affected; the most common signs are:

1. Eye signs – ptosis, diplopia and blurred vision
2. Myasthenic facies
3. Respiratory muscle weakness

These patients may present problems because of:

1. Altered response to anaesthetic drugs especially neuromuscular blocking agents
2. Impaired respiratory function
3. Labile emotional status with anxiety and depression
4. Dysrhythmias due to myocardial involvement

They are normally receiving maintenance anticholinesterase therapy pre-operatively but the effects of anaesthesia and surgery may alter requirements, resulting in either myasthenic or cholinergic crises post-operatively.

In view of the complicated management and careful monitoring required, these patients are usually transferred directly to an intensive care unit after all but the most minor surgery. When they are nursed in the recovery unit, attention must be directed towards:

1. *Maintenance of a clear airway* in the presence of a weak cough reflex and excessive salivation following anticholinesterase therapy
2. *Maintenance of adequate ventilation* with monitoring of neuromuscular transmission and blood gases if necessary
3. *Pain relief.* Small increments of opiates should be given intravenously, with the dose being titrated against the patient's response, if a local anaesthetic block has not been performed
4. *ECG monitoring and the treatment of arrhythmias.* Respiratory inadequacy occurring post-operatively may be due to either an exacerbation of the myasthenia (myasthenic crisis) or a relative overdose of anticholinesterase (cholinergic crisis). Differentiating between the two can sometimes be made by injecting edrophonium 2–4 mg i.v. If there is no improvement or increased weakness, this indicates a cholinergic crisis. However, differentiation may not be straightforward, and adequate ventilatory support must take precedence over attempts at diagnosis.

Muscular Dystrophy

After general anaesthesia patients with dystrophia myotonica will be managed in the intensive care unit with full ventilatory support until normal respiratory function has returned. If they are admitted to the recovery room it must be remembered that they are particularly sensitive to:

1. Suxamethonium (succinylcholine), which may precipitate sustained muscular contractions
2. Neostigmine
3. Barbiturates
4. Opiates

Paraplegia

1. Frequent changes in posture are required to prevent the formation of skin ulcers at pressure areas. Pressure areas must be adequately padded.
2. Changes in posture should be made slowly to prevent hypotension due to autonomic dysfunction.
3. Stimulation below the level of the cord damage (e.g. bladder distension) may lead to an excessive sympathetic discharge, resulting in hypertension, tachycardia and dysrhythmias.
4. Hypothermia is common and intravenous and irrigation fluids require warming.
5. Suxamethonium (succinylcholine) may cause hyperkalaemia with subsequent dysrhythmias or even cardiac arrest if given in the weeks or months immediately after the cord has been damaged. Thereafter, it is safe.

Liver Disease

Liver dysfunction can lead to problems in the recovery room because:

1. *Drug metabolism is decreased.* Patients are unable to tolerate normal drug dosages, which must be reduced accordingly. Of special relevance in the recovery situation are:
   a) Opiates
   b) Local anaesthetics, especially amides, e.g. lignocaine (lidocaine)
   c) Citrate: hypocalcaemia is more likely following blood transfusion
2. *Plasma cholinesterase may be reduced,* causing prolonged neuromuscular block following suxamethonium (succinylcholine). Assisted ventilation must be continued until adequate muscle power has returned.
3. *Reduction of clotting factors.* Factors V, VII, IX and X as well as prothrombin and fibrinogen are synthesised in the liver. Vitamin K deficiency will be a significant contributory factor if there is obstructive jaundice. If

coagulation is impaired, vitamin K (phytonadione) and fresh frozen plasma should be administered. Coagulation studies may be required (see p. 104)

4. *Albumin levels are reduced.*
   a) Diuretics may be required if oedema is significant.
   b) Drugs bound to albumin, e.g. pancuronium, will be potentiated. This may lead to a prolonged action requiring continued ventilatory assistance.

5. *Renal failure.* In patients with obstructive jaundice, conjugated bilirubin renders the kidneys more sensitive to the effects of hypoxia. To prevent renal failure in these patients, a good urine output must be maintained by adequate hydration and the administration of mannitol.

Renal Disease

Severe renal disease may affect a patient's recovery from anaesthesia because of the presence of:

1. *Uraemia,* which may cause tremor, muscle twitching, convulsions, drowsiness and coma.

2. *Impaired urine production.* With the danger of circulatory overload intravenous fluids should be restricted. The use of a Metriset will reduce the possibility of accidental infusion of large volumes. Central venous pressure measurements will provide a useful guide to requirements. A bladder catheter should be inserted.

3. *Hyperkalaemia*, which may cause a characteristic ECG pattern with high peaked T waves. If arrhythmias occur, potassium levels may be reduced by insulin and dextrose. In an emergency calcium may be given to restore the Ca:K ratio.

4. *Acidosis* which may lead to gasping respirations and require treatment with sodium bicarbonate.

5. *Drug excretion is impaired.* Drugs which rely on renal excretion for elimination, such as digoxin and the aminoglycosides, will accumulate and dosages must be reduced accordingly.

6. *Hypertension.* Blood pressure is frequently raised in this condition so that hypertension occurring post-operatively should be interpreted accordingly.

7. *Anaemia*, which is common. Blood loss must be replaced to maintain the patient's usual low haemoglobin concentration. There is no benefit to be gained by attempting to restore the haemoglobin to what is 'normal' for patients without renal failure.

8. *The presence of arteriovenous shunts.* These must be treated with extreme care to avoid the possibility of damage or clotting. Blood pressure readings should not be taken on the same arm as the shunt. Drugs should not be injected through the shunt. Intravenous infusions should not be set up in the same arm as the shunt.

Endocrine Disorders

Diabetes Mellitus

This is a chronic metabolic disease characterised by hyperglycaemia and glycosuria due to insulin deficiency or insensitivity. It is associated with small vessel disease of the kidney, the nervous tissue and the retina.

In the post-operative period, as during anaesthesia, the aim is to prevent:

1. Diabetic ketoacidosis
2. Hypoglycaemia
3. Severe fluid loss

This will be achieved by:

1. *Supportive therapy*
   a) Prevention of hypoxia
   b) Monitoring of vital signs
   c) Assessment of urine output

2. *Intravenous fluid and electrolyte therapy*
   a) 5% dextrose infusion, if the blood glucose level falls below 15 mmol/litre
   b) Dextrose saline (4% dextrose and 0.18% sodium chloride) is an alternative
   c) Regular estimation of the blood glucose may be carried out using Dextrostix and Reflomat. Laboratory estimations of the blood sugar levels at longer intervals should also be undertaken.
   d) The serum potassium level should be checked and kept within normal limits (3.5–5.5 mmol/litre).

3. *Insulin therapy*
   A wide variety of methods of administering insulin are in use. These include:
   a) Low-dose intravenous insulin infusion. Between 4 and 12 units/hour of soluble insulin with a small amount of Haemaccel to prevent absorption of the insulin through the plastic tubing
   b) Regular intramuscular insulin at hourly intervals. Depending on the measured blood sugar level, no insulin may be necessary, and many patients will not require amounts of insulin beyond their normal requirements.

4. *Correction of acidosis*
   The use of bicarbonate to correct any acidosis is probably unnecessary unless the arterial blood pH is less than 7.10–7.15. Acidosis will usually be corrected by insulin and intravenous fluid replacement.

5. *Glycosuria*
   Although a useful sign, levels of glucose in the urine should not now be used to guide management, especially in the early post-operative phase when gross changes in urine osmolality are taking place.

Thyroid Disease

Hypothyroidism

Hypothyroidism may lead to problems including:

1. Prolonged recovery time due to decreased metabolic rate and consequent decreased rate of drug metabolism (see p. 93)
2. Hypothermia in the post-operative period due to loss of normal temperature control (see p. 98)
3. Tracheal deviation and respiratory obstruction if a goitre is present
4. Bradycardia (see p. 83)

Hyperthyroidism

Problems with patients who have hyperthyroidism include:

1. Labile blood pressure, which may require active management (see p. 82)
2. Dysrhythmias (see p. 87)
3. Restlessness (see p. 94)

The problems of a thyrotoxic crisis have been discussed and the management outlined on p. 122.

Phaeochromocytoma

A phaeochromocytoma is a tumour of chromaffin tissue that characteristically produces and excretes excessive amounts of catecholamines. Following incomplete removal there may be further catecholamine release with:

1. α stimulation causing hypertension (see p. 93)
2. β stimulation causing tachycardia (see p. 85) or dysrhythmias (see p. 87)

If removal has been complete, there may be circulatory collapse requiring treatment with intravenous fluids and vasopressors. Steroid cover may be required if adrenalectomy has been performed.

Patients with phaeochromocytomas require continuous arterial pressure measurement and ECG recording and should be transferred directly to an intensive care unit post-operatively.

Porphyria

Porphyria is a rare metabolic disorder characterised by abnormalities of porphyrin metabolism. Serious complications can develop in patients with acute intermittent porphyria, which is exacerbated by the administration of barbiturates and may therefore present in the recovery room.

Features include:

1. Fever, tachycardia and hypertension
2. Acute abdominal pain and vomiting
3. Psychiatric disturbances
4. Muscle paralysis
5. Urine which becomes reddish-brown on standing

An acute attack may require controlled ventilation for a prolonged period and transfer to an intensive care unit will be required. Analgesia is best achieved by regional techniques or opiates. It has been recommended that pentazocine should be avoided.

Haematological Disease

Iron Deficiency Anaemia

Hypoxia must be avoided in patients with iron deficiency anaemia. There is a reduction in the oxygen content of the blood, though not necessarily in the oxygen tension. The oxyhaemoglobin dissociation curve is shifted to the right. Additional inspired oxygen should be given to these patients post-operatively and the anaemia corrected. Patients with stable chronic anaemias tolerate their reduced haemoglobin concentration well and there is little to be gained by attempting to obtain a 'normal' haemoglobin level.

Haemophilia

Haemophilia is an inherited disorder of coagulation caused by reduced levels of factors VIII (true haemophilia) or IX (Christmas disease). It only occurs in males and results in prolonged bleeding following minor trauma. If such patients require surgery, haematological advice should be sought and replacement clotting factors transfused before the operation. The patient's clotting time should be measured regularly post-operatively and further clotting factors given as required.

Many haemophiliacs are carriers of the Human Immunodeficiency Virus (HIV) because they have been given contaminated clotting factors. Their HIV status should be determined before they come to theatre and appropriate precautions taken. In an emergency, when HIV status is not known, they should be assumed to be HIV antigen positive. Newly diagnosed haemophiliacs are not a high risk group as the clotting factors currently used are not contaminated with the virus.

Sickle Cell Disease

Sickle cell disease is a recessive hereditary haemolytic anaemia; it is frequently found in patients of African or West Indian descent, and is due to the replacement of normal haemoglobin by abnormal haemoglobin S. In homozygous sickle cell anaemia, 90% of the haemoglobin is of the S variety. In sickle cell trait (the heterozygous state) less than 40% of the haemoglobin is S. These patients usually present no anaesthetic or recovery room risks.

If the arterial oxygen tension falls below 40 mmHg, the reduced haemoglobin S forms 'tactoids' which distort and rupture the red cells, causing increased plasma viscosity and occlusion of small vessels. The critical level for patients with sickle cell trait is much lower, probably at 20 mmHg. Other variants of sickle cell disease include sickle cell-haemoglobin C disease (SC) and sickle cell-thalassaemia disease. The homozygous patients may have a multiplicity of life-threatening problems due to:

1. Thrombotic lesions in the lungs, kidneys, brain and bones
2. Hepatosplenomegaly
3. Shift of oxyhaemoglobin dissociation curve to the right
4. Cardiomegaly

Prevention of sickling is of paramount importance in the recovery room and management aims to:

1. Prevent hypoxia – administration of oxygen throughout the recovery period.
2. Maintain normothermia
3. Prevent acidosis – administration of sodium bicarbonate if necessary
4. Prevent circulatory stasis – e.g. caused by tourniquets or inadequate peripheral perfusion. The prolonged use of a sphygmomanometer cuff for blood pressure measurement should be avoided. Hypovolaemia and myocardial depression must be prevented

Post-operative anticoagulation may be required to prevent venous thrombosis and pulmonary emboli.

The signs of a sickle cell crisis are:

1. *Vaso-occlusive*: tissue ischaemia
2. *Aplastic*: sudden fall in red cell production leading to weakness and myocardial decompensation
3. *Sequestration*: usually in the spleen, leading to hypovolaemia and shock

Deficiency of Clotting Factors (see p. 104)

Musculoskeletal Disease

Rheumatoid Arthritis

These patients will often appear chronically ill, undernourished and anaemic. They may need to undergo major joint surgery to correct their restrictive deformities.

Problems in the recovery room:

1. *Airway*
   Because of temporo-mandibular joint disease, atlanto-axial subluxation, cervical spine immobility and laryngeal tissue abnormalities, these patients are often extremely hazardous to intubate and the airway may prove difficult to maintain. A nasopharyngeal airway is often very useful.

2. *Pulmonary function*
   A restrictive deformity due to costovertebral joint and vertebral disease may be present, as may diffuse interstitial fibrosis. Blood gas analysis and lung function test should be performed pre-operatively. Care should be exercised when opiate analgesics are used so that respiratory depression does not occur.

3. *Bleeding*
   Chronic anaemia is common and blood loss should be carefully estimated and replaced. Thrombocytopenia may contribute to a coagulopathy.

4. *Steroid therapy*
   Adequate steroid supplementation is vital both pre- and post-operatively as the patient will be unable to produce adequate endogenous steroid to cover the stress of surgery (see p. 145).

5. *Fluid balance*
   Because of rheumatoid renal disease, intravenous fluid replacement will need caution and urine output may require monitoring.

6. *Transit*
   If feasible the patient should be nursed on their bed rather than a trolley, as it will be more comfortable.

Osteoporosis

Care in lifting or transferring these patients is needed to prevent accidental fractures of their weakened bones.

Ankylosing Spondylitis

In this condition, the vertebral joints gradually fuse so that flexion, extension and rotation of the spine become impossible. It may be difficult to maintain a clear airway in these patients, and the insertion of a nasopharyngeal airway until they are fully conscious will help. The neck may be fixed in a position of flexion and pillows should be adjusted accordingly.

Geriatric Patients

The geriatric patient will present many physiological and psychological problems in the recovery room.

1. *Cardiovascular*
   a) Decreased myocardial reserve
   b) Coronary artery disease
   c) Increased susceptibility to dysrhythmias
   d) Decreased cardiac output
   Hypotension leading to decrease in oxygen transport must be avoided, as must hypertension, which may lead to cerebrovascular haemorrhage.
2. *Respiration*
   a) Decreased lung compliance
   b) Decrease in vital capacity and total lung capacity
   c) Increased shunting
   All these factors will lead to an increased degree of hypoxia and hypercarbia in the geriatric post-operative patient.
   Secretions should be cleared and chest infections prevented by early physiotherapy. The sitting position will aid ventilation although this may prove difficult in the arthritic patient with multiple bony deformities.
3. *Anaemia*
   These patients are often chronically anaemic and the prevention of respiratory obstruction and hypoxia is thus particularly important.
4. *Renal function*
   Drug eliminiation may be slow. Fluid retention and drug accumulation can occur and should be considered when managing the post-operative fluid and analgesic regime.
5. *Skin Care*
   It is obviously very important to prevent bed sores when the skin is fragile and slow to heal.
6. *Confusion*
   Every effort should be made to guide these patients through the recovery time without subjecting them to undue anxiety or tension.
7. *Hypothermia*
   Loss of subcutaneous fat allows heat loss whilst a reduced muscle mass reduces the value of shivering as a source of heat production.

Pregnancy

Post-operative recovery room care for this group of patients includes:

1. Prevention of hypoxia; oxygen should be given
2. Prevention of hypovolaemia and hypotension
3. Adequate analgesia and sedation
4. In late pregnancy the patient should be nursed in the left lateral position, thus preventing the possibility of vena caval obstruction, which may lead to maternal hypotension and fetal hypoxia and acidosis.

These patients may require reassurance concerning the safety of the unborn child.

Malnourishment

Special attention must be paid to preventing pressure sores in malnourished patients. Frequent turning will be required if there is a prolonged stay in the recovery unit as trolleys are notoriously firm. Alternatively, the patient may be nursed on a bed. Intramuscular injections are particularly painful as an appropriate muscle mass may be impossible to find. Intravenous or subcutaneous routes are suitable alternatives.

The malnourished are sensitive to many drugs as less drug will be bound to albumin and globulin and more will be unbound and active. Dosages must be reduced accordingly.

Intravenous feeding may be in progress via a central venous line. Drugs should not be injected into that line nor should it be used for obtaining blood samples.

In severe malnutrition, plasma cholinesterase levels will be low and prolonged neuromuscular block may follow suxamethonium (succinylcholine) administration so that ventilatory assistance may be required (see p. 73).

Obesity

1. *Airway maintenance* requires careful attention, especially in the patient with a short thick neck.
2. *Ventilation* is impaired by the weight of abdominal contents pressing on the diaphragm, splinting its movements. Atelectasis is common especially after upper abdominal procedures and results in shunting and an increased alveolar-arterial oxygen pressure difference. The following prove helpful:
   a) Oxygen by face mask to increase F_1O_2

b) Sitting the patient up to lessen pressure on the diaphragm as soon as consciousness returns

c) Pain relief by epidural or other local anaesthetic block as appropriate

d) Physiotherapy to encourage deep breathing

Progress can be monitored by comparing serial blood gases with pre-operative baseline values. A period of elective ventilation may be required. Extubation should not be performed until ventilatory function is satisfactory.

3. *Deep vein thrombosis* is more common in the obese patient and early mobilisation should be encouraged. Prophylactic heparinisation is frequently used.

4. *Moving and lifting* patients is difficult and should not be attempted without adequate help.

5. *Venous lines* must be carefully preserved since replacement may be impossible without a cut down.

6. *Blood pressure estimations* by indirect methods are difficult to obtain and the correct sized cuff must be used (Table 2.3). Hypertension is common in the obese. Arterial cannulation may be the most satisfactory method of obtaining accurate readings.

Further Reading

Albert KGMM, Thomas DJB (1979) The management of diabetes during surgery. Br J Anaesth 51: 693–710

Aldrete JA, Guerra F (1981) Hematological disease. In: Katz J, Benumof J, Kadis LB (eds) Anaesthesia and uncommon diseases, WB Saunders, Philadelphia, pp. 313–383

Bevan DR (1979) Renal function in anaesthesia and surgery. Academic Press, London

Caldwell TB (1981) Anaesthesia for patients with behavioral and environmental disorders. In: Katz J, Benumof J, Kadis LB (eds) Anaesthesia and uncommon diseases. WB Saunders, Philadelphia pp 672–777

Chung DC (1982) Anaesthesia in patients with ischaemic heart disease. Edward Arnold, London

Davenport H (1986) Anaesthesia in the elderly. Heinemann Medical Books, London

Fisher A, Waterhouse TD, Adams AP (1975) Obesity: its relation to anaesthesia. Anaesthesia 30: 633–647

Foëx P (1981) Preoperative assessment of the patient with cardiovascular disease. Br J Anaesth 53: 731–744

Fox GS, Whalley DG, Bevan DR (1981) Anaesthesia for the morbidly obese: experience with 110 patients. Br J Anaesth 53: 811–816

Gareth J (1982) Symposium on anaesthesia and respiratory function. Br J Anaesth 54: 701–782

Goldman L, Caldera DL, Nussbaum SR et al. (1977) Multifactorial index of cardiac risk in noncardiac surgical procedures. N Engl J Med 297: 845–850

Gothard JWW (1987) Anaesthesia for cardiac surgery and allied procedures. Blackwell Scientific Publications, Oxford

Leventhal SR, Orkin FK, Hirsh RA (1980) Prediction for the need for postoperative mechanical ventilation in myasthenia gravis. Anaesthesiology 53: 26–30

Marshall A J (1981) Drug therapy of hypertension and ischaemic heart disease. Br J Anaesth 53: 697–710

Prys-Roberts CPR (1980) The circulation in anaesthesia. Blackwell Scientific Publications, Oxford

Strunin L (1977) The liver and anaesthesia. Butterworths, London

Sykes MK, McNicol MW, Campbell EJM (1976) Respiratory failure. Blackwell Scientific Publications, Oxford
Taylor TH, Major E (1987) Hazards and complications of anaesthesia. Churchill Livingstone, London
Vickers MD (1982) Medicine for anaesthetists. Blackwell Scientific Publications, Oxford
Vickers MD, Wood-Smith FG, Stewart HC (1978) Drugs in anaesthetic practice. Butterworths, London
Watkins J Salo M (1982) Trauma, stress and immunity in anaesthesia and surgery. Butterworth Scientific, London

Chapter 7

Recovery and Day Surgery

Day surgery is not new but in recent years it has become seen as an economically efficient method of performing uncomplicated surgery and so reducing hospital waiting lists. Patients may be admitted to either a free-standing day surgery unit or to the in-patient wards. However, if patient safety is not to be compromised, strict guidelines should be formulated and observed.

Patient Selection

Not all patients are suitable for day surgery. Selection criteria will vary from unit to unit. Relevant factors include:

1. The patient must be accompanied home by a responsible adult who should remain available until the following day.
2. The patient must be under 70 years of age.
3. The patient should live within a 20 mile radius of the hospital.
4. The patient should be generally fit and well.
5. Patient should not eat or drink for 6 h before general anaesthesia.
6. Surgery should not be expected to last longer than 30 min.
7. The operation should not be expected to produce severe post-operative pain or bleeding.

Procedures Suitable for Day Surgery

A wide range of procedures in many specialties can be safely carried out on day stay patients:

General Surgery

Excision of cysts and lipomata
Ligation of varicose veins
Removal of in-growing toenails
Herniorrhaphy
Anal dilatation
Cystoscopy, gastroscopy, colonoscopy
Vasectomy
Circumcision

Gynaecology

Dilatation and curettage
Termination of pregnancy
Laparoscopy
Tubal ligation
Excision of Bartholin's cyst

Orthopaedics

Arthroscopy
Excision of ganglia
Carpal tunnel decompression
Trigger finger release
Removal of screws
Manipulation under anaesthesia

Ear, Nose and Throat (ENT)

Endoscopies
Myringotomy
Insertion of grommets
Antral lavage
Reduction of fractured nasal bones

Dentistry

Dental extraction
Dental conservation in the mentally handicapped
Apicectomy

Pain Clinic Procedures

Nerve blocks
Sympathectomies
I.V. guanethidine blocks

Documentation

It is extremely useful for all day stay patients to complete a standard question-naire. This should not only cover their general health but also confirm that they have not eaten for 6 h, will be accompanied home and will have assistance immediately to hand at home. Such a chart will also enable the recovery unit nurse to quickly spot any areas that may give rise to problems after surgery.

The patient questionnaire should contain a clear statement that it is danger-ous to drive, ride a bicycle or operate machinery (including cookers) for 24 h after a general anaesthetic.

Anaesthetic Techniques

Premedication is rarely offered to day surgery patients as it tends to prolong recovery. A sympathetic explanation of what is to be done to them will help allay their natural anxiety.

If general anaesthesia is used, agents that are rapidly metabolised and excreted should be used. Propofol is probably the induction agent of choice and isoflurane may be the best volatile agent to use. Effective intra-operative analgesia can be obtained with fentanyl which tends not to cause prolonged post-operative somnolence. If intubation is required, suxamethonium is a suitable relaxant.

Benzodiazepines (diazepam or midazolam) are often used for sedating patients undergoing dental surgery or endoscopies. Although patients may appear fully recovered after such sedation, they often suffer from a considerable degree of amnesia.

Nausea and vomiting are infrequent after modern anaesthesia but possibly occur more frequently in day stay patients who are ambulant soon after their operation. A suitable anti-emetic should be prescribed and administered as necessary. Drowsiness and headaches are the other problems which patients encounter most commonly.

Regional anaesthetic techniques (see p. 142) are especially valuable for day surgery as they do not produce these side-effects and additionally provide useful post-operative analgesia. Many of the orthopaedic and general surgical procedures suitable for day surgery can easily be performed after a local anaesthetic block. A combination of a local anaesthetic block and a general anaesthetic may be the ideal for other procedures such as circumcision in children.

Recovery from Anaesthesia

Day stay patients should be nursed as they recover from their anaesthetic in exactly the same way as all other patients (see Chap. 2). They should be positioned appropriately, given oxygen, and have their vital signs monitored and recorded. Their recovery, however, is likely to be uncomplicated and consciousness should return rapidly if they have been cared for by a competent anaesthetist. They are unlikely to have required an i.v. infusion or to have any surgical drains or tubes in place. Any pain, nausea or vomiting should be quickly treated.

Once they are fully conscious and their condition stable, arrangements should be made for them to have a drink and something to eat. This is especially important for children who do not understand why they are being starved.

Discharge from the Day Unit

Numerous tests have been described that seek to determine when a patient is sufficiently recovered to be discharged. No single test is ideal or a substitute for a careful clinical evaluation.

Before patients are discharged from the recovery area and allowed to go home, the following criteria must be fulfilled:

1. The patient must be able to dress and care for himself.
2. The patient must be accompanied home by a responsible adult who will remain available for 24 h.
3. The patient must be warned verbally and in writing against driving or operating any form of machinery for 24 h. As short-term memory is impaired after anaesthesia and benzodiazepine sedation, the written warning is especially important.
4. The patient should be pain free and suitable oral analgesics should be provided to take should pain return.
5. The wound should be inspected and, if necessary, dressings should be provided.
6. The patient should be told who to contact if unexpected post-operative problems arise.
7. Arrangements for follow-up care, the removal of stitches etc. should be confirmed.

No patients should be discharged if they feel unwell or if their escorts are unhappy to take responsibility for them. Facilities should always be available to admit day stay patients if surgical complications have been encountered or if their general condition precludes their safe discharge.

Post-anaesthetic Complications

Anaesthetic complications that ordinarily are seen and treated routinely on an in-patient ward can be considered extremely worrying when they occur in a day stay patient who has returned home. It is very valuable if patients are warned of the commoner problems that may occur and given information about who to contact if a problem persists.

Most anaesthetic complications are minor and self-limiting and explanation and reassurance are usually the only treatment that is necessary.

Regional or Local Anaesthesia

Pain or 'pins and needles' will occur as any local anaesthetic block wears off. Backache can be caused by minor local trauma that occurs when epidurals or sympathectomies are performed. Patients should be given oral analgesia as sensation returns.

Hypotension can occur after epidural or caudal blocks because of sympathetically mediated vasodilatation. It may manifest itself as dizziness on standing or lightheadedness. Patients should be advised to avoid sudden changes in posture and encouraged to take oral fluids.

Motor blockade can be very worrying if it persists. Patients can be reassured that it rarely lasts longer than 4–6 h. They should also be warned of the potential problem of a partially blocked leg giving way or a partially blocked arm dropping suddenly to their side.

Retention of urine can follow epidural or caudal blocks. It is wise to ensure that patients have passed urine before allowing them home.

General Anaesthesia

Drowsiness, nausea and vomiting have been considered above.

Hangover is probably the commonest side-effect of general anaesthesia. Although patients may appear to recover quickly and completely, they will tend to be below par for 24–48 h after a general anaesthetic. Patients with domestic responsibilities who attempt to run their homes without help are likely to suffer most.

Sore throats are traditionally blamed on oral intubation but occur almost as frequently in patients who are not intubated. They may be due to breathing dry anaesthetic gases or to the use of oral airways. They rarely last longer than 24–48 h and may be helped by gargles.

Muscular aches and pains may occur if suxamethonium (succinylcholine) is used prior to intubation. They particularly affect the shoulder girdle muscles and are said to be more frequent and severe in fit young patients who mobilise early. There is no specific treatment but simple analgesics may help. Non-specific aches and pains may occur in patients who have not had suxamethonium. They may be due to the position in which the patient had lain when on the operating table. If there is pain or weakness in the distribution of a specific nerve or nerve plexus, the degree of deficit should be carefully recorded and appropriate follow-up management arranged. Most deficits are neuropraxias and will recover spontaneously.

Bruising may occur at injection sites but needs no specific treatment. If thrombophlebitis occurs, non-steroidal anti-inflammatory agents may help relieve discomfort.

Visual disturbances can be due to the residual effects of general anaesthesia and recover spontaneously. A sensation of grittiness in the eye will probably be due to corneal drying when the eye-lids have not been closed during anaesthesia. Foreign bodies must be excluded if prompt recovery does not occur.

Most of these problems are annoying rather than dangerous. Patients can have most of their natural anxieties relieved by careful explanation and by giving them a telephone number they can ring for further advice.

Further Reading

Burn JMB (1979) A blue print for day surgery. Anaesthesia 34: 790–805

Gould JE (1983) Anaesthesia for day care surgery: a review. J Roy Soc Med 76: 415–420

Kalmanovitch DVA, Simmons P (1988) Post-anaesthetic complications in the home. Prescriber's Journal 28: 124–131

Ogg TW (1980) Use of anaesthesia: implications of day case surgery and anaesthesia. BMJ 2: 212–214

Ogg TW (1985) Aspects of day surgery and anaesthesia. Anaesthesia Rounds, Pharmaceutical Division, ICI, England

Chapter 8

Monitoring

All efforts which are made to detect problems early in the vital post-operative recovery period should decrease patient morbidity and mortality. Monitoring is the process whereby systematic observation and subsequent evaluation occur so that actual or potential changes in a patient's physiological state may be quickly recognised. Appropriate treatment can then be initiated. Patient monitoring must, thus, be a continuous decision-making process. It requires data to be collected and the collector to have sufficient knowledge to interpret and act on those data. Care must be taken, however, to ensure that staff are not submerged by excessive amounts of new data and so miss vital changes in the clinical state of the patient. Observing the patient must remain paramount.

In the recovery area, part of the nurse's role will be to collect and organise data so as to define a particular patient's status. This will often result in situations where the nurse will also interpret data and initiate therapy without referring to a doctor. In other circumstances it will be more appropriate to seek medical advice.

In the early post-operative phase, monitoring is mainly directed towards the detection of complications of recovery from anaesthesia. The degree and sophistication of monitoring will depend on the specific needs of the patient. These needs will be determined by a number of factors including age, anaesthetic risk, metabolic state, pre-existing cardiovascular or respiratory disease, and the often overlooked surgical procedure that has been carried out and the primary disease which had made surgery necessary.

Much work has been carried out to determine what is the most appropriate level of monitoring for a given patient and it appears that three levels of monitoring are necessary:

1. Routine or standard
2. Advanced or special
3. Intensive or highly sophisticated

This last category would be appropriate for those patients who are at high risk of multi-organ failure because of pre-existing disease or surgical intervention. The recovery room should be able to provide either standard or advanced monitoring. Invasive and intensive monitoring are more the domain of intensive care of high dependancy units.

ASA Classification

The degree of risk for each individual patient must be determined and the appropriate levels of monitoring then provided. Many different techniques of 'risk audit' are now available. Probably the most simple and useful is that proposed by the American Society of Anaesthesiologists (ASA) (Table 8.1):

ASA 1 can be monitored basically.

ASA 2 and 3 will require a more advanced level of monitoring.

ASA 4 and 5 will require more advanced monitoring and most probably transfer into an intensive monitoring environment such as the Intensive Care Unit.

Table 8.1. Physical status classification of the American Society of Anesthesiologists (ASA) adapted from Anesthesiology (1963) 24: 111

Status	Disease state
ASA Class 1	No organic, physiological, biochemical, or psychiatric disturbance
ASA Class 2	Mild to moderate systemic disturbance that may or may not be related to the reason for surgery; e.g. heart disease that only slightly limits physical activity, essential hypertension, diabetes mellitus, anaemia, extremes of age, morbid obesity, chronic bronchitis
ASA Class 3	Severe systemic disturbance that may or may not be related to the reason of surgery; e.g. heart disease that limits activity, poorly controlled essential hypertension, diabetes mellitus with vascular complications, chronic pulmonary disease that limits activity, angina pectoris, history of prior myocardial infarction
ASA Class 4	Severe systemic disturbance that is life-threatening with or without surgery; e.g. congestive heart failure, persistent angina pectoris, advanced pulmonary, renal, or hepatic dysfunction
ASA Class 5	Moribund patient who has little chance of survival with or without surgery; e.g. uncontrolled haemorrhage from a ruptured abdominal aneurysm, major cerebral trauma, major pulmonary embolus
Emergency (E)	Any patient in whom an emergency operation is required; e.g. an otherwise healthy 30-year old female who requires a dilatation and currettage for moderate but persistent haemorrhage (ASA Class 1 E)

Routine Monitoring

This is the usual level of monitoring and can be considered as an extension of routine physical examination which should follow the usual format of such as examination:

1. Inspection
2. Palpation
3. Percussion
4. Auscultation

For example, one will inspect:

The skin and nail beds for colour and capillary refill

The mucous membranes for colour and, more importantly, for the degree of dryness or moisture

The surgical site for swelling or rate of blood loss

Movement, to note whether or not it is a purposeful response to a stimulus such as pain or speech

Palpation will be used to feel for skin temperature, muscle tone and the volume, rate and regularity of the pulse. *Percussion* may be used to determine the degree of gastric distension or of bladder filling. *Auscultation* is most commonly employed in the measurement of blood pressure with a sphygnomanometer.

Respiratory System

The most fundamental observations of respiratory function are:

1. *Colour, central and peripheral.*
2. *Respiratory rate and degree of respiratory effort.* Further, respiratory parameters that could be measured in the recovery room include tidal volume (V_t), peak expiratory flow rate (PEFR), and forced expiratory volume (FEV_1).
3. *Carbon dioxide tension using:*
   a) Blood gas analysis
   b) Transcutaneous CO_2 tension electrodes
   c) Capnography
4. *Oxygen tension* using:
   a) Blood gas analysis
   b) Transcutaneous oxygen tension electrodes
5. *Oxygen saturation* using:
   a) A pulse oximeter with the probe on an ear or finger or, in the case of neonates and infants, across the palm of a hand or the sole of a foot.
   b) The measurement of mixed venous oxygen saturation in blood taken from a central venous or pulmonary artery catheter.

Post-operative lung ventilation may, on occasion, be required in the recovery room. It is then necessary to have the facility to measure certain aspects of lung mechanics. These will include:

Expired lung volumes

Peak airway pressures

Positive and expiratory pressure (PEEP)
Airway compliance and resistance

A chest X-ray may often complement the above information especially if a pneumothorax may have occurred following either the insertion of a central venous line or surgery in the neck or near the diaphragm.

Cardiovascular System

Routine measurement of haemodynamic parameters should include:

1. Heart rate
2. Blood pressure
3. Urine output
4. Temperature

There should also be facilities to monitor:

1. Electrocardiogram
2. Blood pressure directly by an arterial line
3. Central venous pressure
4. Pulmonary artery pressure
5. Cardiac output

Although not routine, the facility to measure these last two parameters should be available and may be useful in the early post-operative management of critically ill patients prior to transfer from the recovery room to the intensive care unit.

Metabolic Systems

The monitoring of these variables will allow for correction of fluid, electrolyte and acid-base abnormalities. It is thus important to measure:

1. Serum electrolytes including sodium, potassium, magnesium and calcium
2. Blood sugar
3. Arterial blood pH and bicarbonate
4. Serum osmolality
5. Serum urea and creatinine
6. Urine osmolality

Neurological System

Although neurological monitoring is largely clinically based using the Glasgow Coma Scale (see p. 126), it is now possible to use more sophisticated and advanced monitoring techniques in the recovery room. These may be of particular value following carotid artery surgery, neurosurgery and orthopaedic surgery involving the vertebral column and spinal cord.

The electroencephalogram (EEG) detects electrical signals from cortical neurones but is often difficult to use as it requires skilled technical interpretation.

The cerebral function monitor is a modified and simplified EEG. There electrodes are placed on the scalp to provide what is known as an integrated EEG whereby the voltage generated by EEG signals has been rectified and amplified. Although providing information on the quantity of electrical activity in the brain, this monitor lacks the specificity that is particularly needed following carotid artery surgery.

Compressed spectral array. Using scalp electrodes, this technique presents a histogram of power and frequency change across the range of EEG signals. The EEG frequencies and power are shown in a graphical display on a VDU and changes with time can be clearly seen. Again, this technique is unable to show changes in specific brain areas.

Evoked potentials. These are wave forms generated by the brain in response to specific stimuli. A *somatosensory evoked potential* (SEP) follows stimulation of a peripheral nerve and may provide information on the functioning of the posterior columns of the cord, the brain stem and cerebral cortex.

Brain stem auditory evoked potentials (BAEP). Auditory signals may be used to test the eighth cranial nerve and provide further information on the functioning of the brain stem and auditory cortex.

Visual evoked potentials (VEP) use light as the stimulus and the areas assessed will be the occipital cortex, lateral geniculate body and cerebral hemispheres. This path obviously does not include the brain stem.

Intracranial pressure (ICP) monitoring will occasionally be used following neurosurgery and as part of the management of a patient who has had major trauma to the cranium.

Specific Monitors

Electrocardiograph (ECG)

An ECG is a graphical representation of variation of cardiac electrical potentials. It is the sum of all the currents flowing through the heart at a given moment and represents the electrical potential of the heart. A systematic approach to analysing the ECG is not beyond the role of recovery room personnel. If the ECG is routinely monitored in the recovery room, expertise will soon be acquired in recognising the commoner abnormalities.

The standard ECG leads are bipolar, that is, they record the potential difference between successive pairs of electrodes. They are most useful in the detection of dysrhythmias, conduction blocks, electrolyte disturbances and myocardial ischaemia.

Lead 1 connects the right arm and left arm electrodes;
Lead 2 connects the right arm and left leg electrodes;
Lead 3 connects the left arm and left leg electrodes.

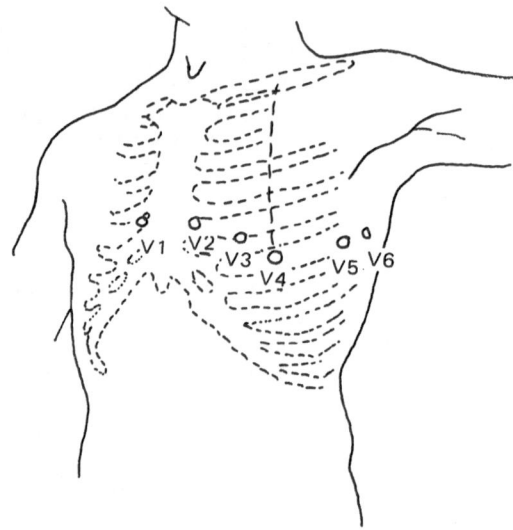

Fig. 8.1.   Precordial polar leads.

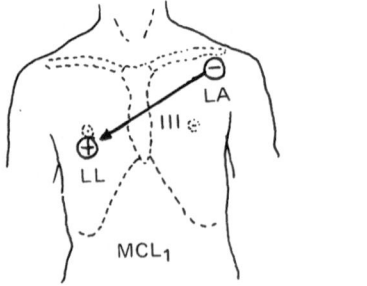
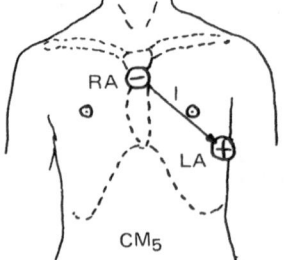

Fig. 8.2.   Modified bipolar standard limb lead systems.

An extension of this bipolar system is the unipolar technique when the three standard leads are used as a common electrode with no potential difference between them. If this is combined with a further active electrode, potential difference between them represents the actual potential. Thus, the unipolar lead system has a neutral electrode formed by the standard leads and an additional electrode termed the 'exploring electrode'. The precordial leads are designated by a letter V plus a numeral corresponding to the location of the electrode on the chest wall. These can be summarised as:

V1. Fourth intercostal space, right sternal edge.
V2. Fourth intercostal space, left sternal edge.
V3. Between V2 and V4.
V4. Fifth intercostal space, mid-clavicular line.
V5. Lateral to V4 in anterior axillary line.
V6. Lateral to V5 in mid-axillary line. (See Fig 8.1.)

The chest leads are useful in interpreting:

Changes in the rotational axis of the heart.
Ventricular hypertrophy.
Bundle branch blocks.
Antero-septal and lateral myocardial ischaemia.

A further extension of this system is the modified bipolar standard lead e.g. CM_5. C suggests that the negative electrode is central, M that the positive electrode position has been modified and 5 that the position of this M lead is at V5. Thus the negative right arm electrode is placed on the sternum, the positive left arm lead in the V5 position and the ground (or left leg) electrode in its usual left leg position. This system is particularly useful for monitoring myocardial ischaemia. For monitoring cardiac rhythm, the system MCL_1 is probably of most use (see Fig. 8.2).

Arterial Pressure

Arterial pressure may be measured by invasive or non-invasive techniques.
Invasive methods. These will give continuous pressure measurements on a beat to beat basis and will also allow easy blood sampling for acid-base, blood gas, electrolyte and haematological measurement and analysis. The site of cannulation is most often the radial, brachial or dorsalis pedis arteries.
Non-invasive methods. These include the use of Doppler ultrasound transducers and oscillotonometry. Oscillotonometric techniques measure blood pressure and heart rate by means of an inflatable cuff. The cuff inflates to occlude an artery and then begins to deflate in a series of increments. As it does so, the monitor will measure the amplitude of the oscillations induced in the cuff by the movement of the arterial wall. A microprocessor within the monitor will then process and store two consecutive pulsations that have equal amplitude and frequency. At each incremental pressure level, the device stores the cuff pressure, pulsation amplitude and the time between successive heartbeats. Using these variables the monitor notes the pressures when pulsations increase, peak and decrease and thus determines systolic, mean and diastolic blood pressures and heart rate. Many such devices are now available which will non-invasively

record blood pressure and heart rate at predetermined intervals. However, the increased use of microprocessor technology has led to the development of many fully integrated devices which will measure and monitor ECG, blood pressure, invasively and non-invasively, oxygen saturation using an oximeter (see p. 176) and carbon dioxide tension using capnography (see p. 177).

Pulmonary Artery Pressure

When patients are critically ill, the measurement of pulmonary artery pressures using a flow-directed balloon-tipped catheter is often indicated. ECG and pressure wave form monitoring are needed when a pulmonary artery catheter is being introduced and full resuscitation equipment should be nearby. The catheter is inserted percutaneously into a central vein and the balloon at its tip inflated. The catheter is carried forward by the blood flow and floats through the right atrium into the right ventricle and then through the pulmonary artery. Once in the main trunk of the pulmonary artery, it will then float out into the right or left pulmonary artery and will continue until it wedges in a distal branch. The balloon is then deflated and the catheter now measures pulmonary artery pressure. When inflated, the balloon will occlude the distal branch of the

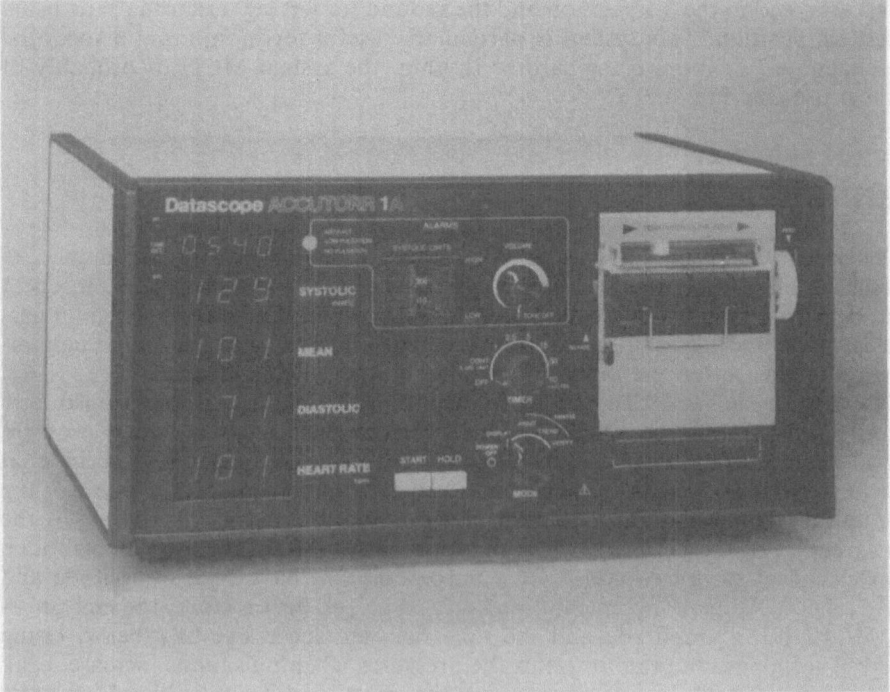

Fig. 8.3. Automated non-invasive blood pressure monitor.

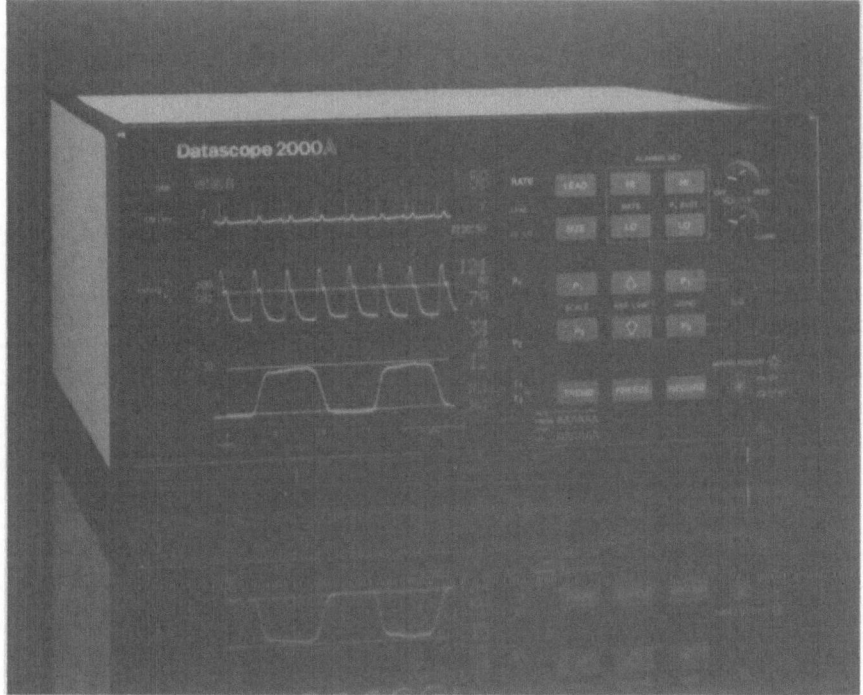

Fig. 8.4. Integrated monitoring system; ECG, invasive blood pressure, temperature and capnography.

pulmonary artery and will measure pulmonary capillary wedge pressure (PCWP). Wedge pressure reflects transmitted pulmonary venous pressure which approximates left atrial pressure. The left atrial pressure, if the left ventricle is normal, will be the left ventricular end diastolic pressure (LVEDP). The normal PCWP ranges from 6–15 mmHg.

It is possible to use a pulmonary artery catheter to measure cardiac output by:

1. The thermodilution technique
2. Dye dilution technique

If the thermodilution technique is to be used, a triple lumen catheter is inserted, with a thermistor near its tip and an extra proximal lumen opening into the right atrium. A 10 ml bolus of saline at 0 °C is injected into the right atrium. It will mix with blood already there and the transient decrease in blood temperature will be detected by the thermistor lying in the pulmonary artery. From a knowledge of the volume and temperature of the cold saline injected into the right atrium and the subsequent drop in temperature in the pulmonary artery, a cardiac output microprocessor will determine the cardiac output.

Oxygen saturation

Prior to the availability of the oximeter, absence of cyanosis was taken as an indication that oxygenation was adequate. Changes in the colour of haemoglobin (Hb) with different degrees of oxygenation have been measured for many years. Recent developments now allow these to be measured accurately and non-invasively utilising the technique of pulse oximetry.

The amount of red light absorbed by Hb varies with its oxygen saturation while the absorption of light of other wavelengths is not altered. Current oximeters send light of several different wavelengths through tissue. The amount of light of all wavelengths received by the detector will depend on the thickness of the tissue and the total amount of Hb present. In addition, the amount of red light received will depend on the degree of Hb oxygen saturation. A microprocessor derives the Hb oxygen saturation from the amount of light detected. The microprocessor is also programmed to record only the saturation

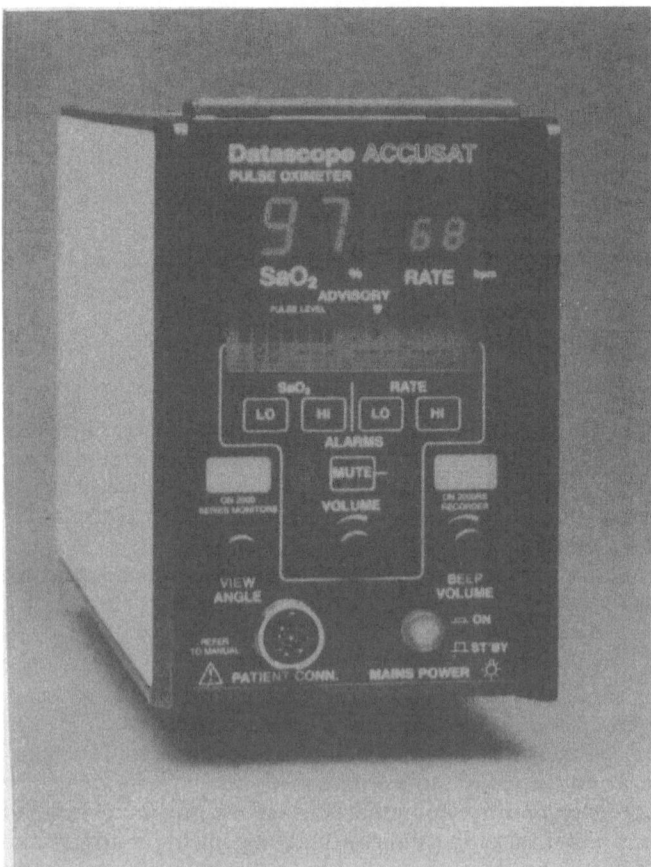

Fig. 8.5. Pulse oximeter.

of Hb that is in pulsating arteries and to disregard that in non-pulsatile veins. Hence, pulse oximeters display the arterial oxygen saturation and not the total Hb oxygen saturation.

The pulse oximeter is designed to be insensitive to haemodynamic changes although extreme hypotension or vasoconstriction may produce a signal too weak for the oximeter to detect. Pulse oximeters are simple to use and non-invasively give continuous information on the degree of arterial oxygenation. Although they represent a significant advance in non-invasive monitoring, they can be inaccurate in the presence of carboxyhaemoglobin, methaemoglobin and fetal haemoglobin or in jaundiced patients.

Neuromuscular Blockade

It may be necessary to monitor neuromuscular blockade to ensure that recovery from muscle relaxants is complete. Many studies have indicated that patients are all too frequently returned to the recovery room partially paralysed. Routine monitoring with a peripheral nerve stimulator makes it possible to achieve precise individual dosing of both muscle relaxants and their antagonists. Some patients have been found to respond in an unpredictable manner to muscle relaxants and therefore monitoring with a peripheral nerve stimulator (PNS) is essential. These include:

1. Patients with a reduced ability to metabolise muscle relaxants e.g. those with liver and renal disease.
2. Debilitated patients with reduced muscle mass.
3. Patients with neuromuscular disease.
4. Morbidly obese patients.
5. Patients during prolonged surgery.

Whatever particular PNS machine is used it should have the ability to administer:

1. A single twitch.
2. A tetanic stimulus of 50–100 Hz.
3. Train-of-four (TOF) stimulation.

TOF stimulation is the application of four supramaximal stimuli (2 Hz) at intervals of 0.5 s over a period of 2 seconds. A patient may be considered to have recovered from the effects of neuromuscular blockers if he shows no evidence of fade on tetanic stimulation and the fourth stimulus in a TOF produces a response that is at least 75% that of the first. The most commonly stimulated peripheral nerves are the median and ulnar nerves.

Carbon Dioxide Tension

The amount of carbon dioxide in expired air can be measured by a capnometer. This transmits a beam of infra-red light through a chamber into which expired

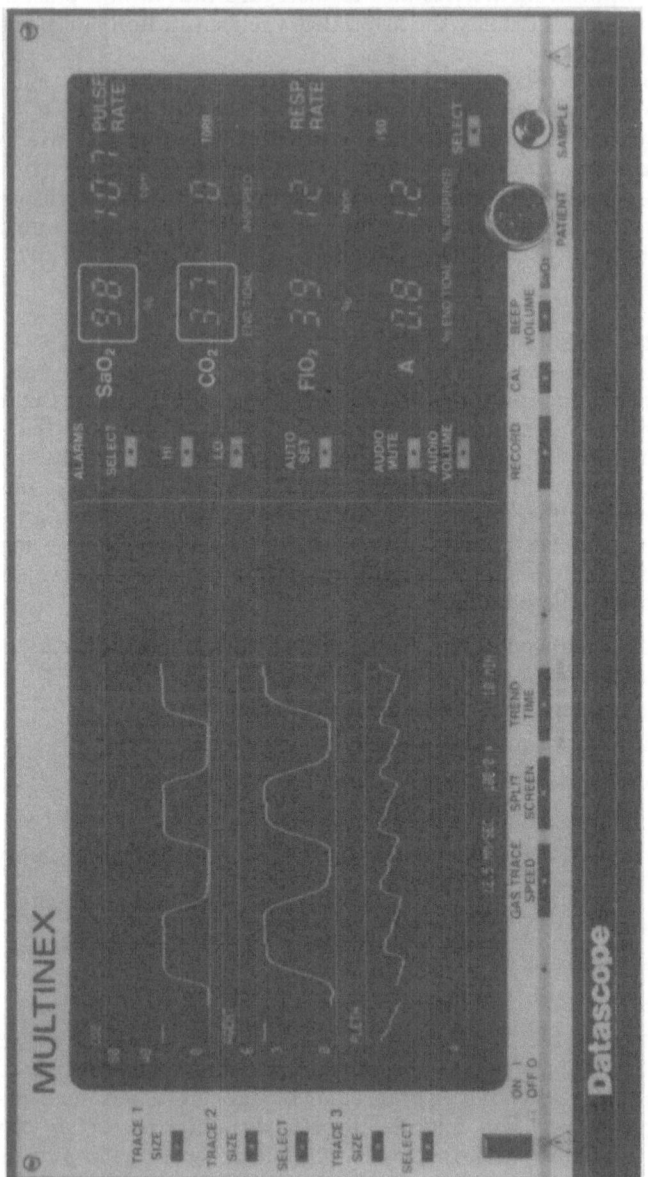

Fig. 8.6. Integrated capnograph, oximeter and inspired oxygen analyser.

air is constantly drawn. The amount of infra-red light absorbed will depend on the amount of carbon dioxide present. Inspired room air can be assumed to contain no CO_2 whereas a normal end tidal CO_2 will be between 4.5% and 5.5%. The measurement of end tidal CO_2 is useful:

1. As an indicator of the adequacy of ventilation in either the spontaneously breathing or ventilated patient.
2. To monitor the adequacy of cardiac output and blood pressure. This is particularly important following the use of induced hypotension when end tidal CO_2 may fall as less CO_2 is being produced. When normal blood pressure and cardiac output are restored there should be an appropriate rise in end tidal CO_2.
3. As an early warning of a venous air embolism. This results in micro-bubbles of air filling the pulmonary vasculature. This will produce a ventilation/perfusion mismatch with retention of CO_2 in the tissues and a consequent fall in expired CO_2.
4. As a ventilator disconnection alarm. A sudden fall in end tidal CO_2 will suggest that the patient has become disconnected from the ventilator.

Further Reading

Blitt CD (1985) Maintaining in anaesthesia and critical care medicine. Churchill Livingstone, London

Gravenstein JS, Newbower RS et al. (1983) An integrated approach to monitoring. Butterworths, London

Lawrence J, Saidman N, Smith T (1984) Maintaining anaesthesia, 2nd ed. Butterworths, London

Macintosh R, Mushin WW, Epstein HG (1987) Physics for the anaesthetist, 4th edn. Blackwell Scientific Publications, Oxford

Sykes MK, Vickers MD, Hull CJ (1981) Principles of clinical measurement, 2nd edn. Blackwell Scientific Publications, Oxford

Taylor TH, Major E (1988) Hazards and complications of anaesthesia. Churchill Livingstone, London

Appendix A. Drugs Commonly Used in a Recovery Room

British name	American name	Effects
Adrenaline	Epinephrine	Positive inotrope, vasopressor
Alcuronium (Alloferin)	Not available	Muscle relaxant
Aminocaproic acid (Epsikapron)	Aminocaproic acid (Amicar)	Anti-fibrinolysis
Aminophylline	Aminophylline (Theophylline)	Bronchodilator
Ampicillin (Penbritin, Amfipen)	Ampicillin (Amcil, Omnipen, Polycillin)	Antibiotic
Aprotinin (Trasylol)	Not available	Trypsin inactivation
Aspirin	Aspirin	Analgesic
Atenolol (Tenormin)	Atenolol (Tenormin)	β-blocker
Atracurium (Tracrium)	Atracurium (Tracrium)	Muscle relaxant
Atropine	Atropine	Anticholinergic
Bupivacaine (Marcain)	Bupivacaine (Marcaine)	Local anaesthetic
Buprenorphine (Temgesic)	Not available	Analgesic
Bumetanide (Burinex)	Bumetanide (Bumex)	Diuretic
Calcium chloride/gluconate	Calcium chloride/gluconate	Inotrope, replacement of Ca^{++}
Cefuroxime (Zinacef)	Cefuroxime (Zinacef)	Antibiotic
Chlormethiazole (Heminevrin)	Not available	Sedative
Chlorpheniramine (Piriton)	Chlorpheniramine (Chlortrimetron, Teldrin)	Antihistamine
Chlorpromazine (Largactil)	Chlorpromazine (Thorazine)	Sedative, antihistamine, α-blocker
Codeine phosphate	Codeine	Analgesic
Dantrolene (Dantrium)	Dantrolene (Dantrium)	Inhibits malignant hyperpyrexia
Deslanoside (Cedilanid)	Deslanoside (Cedilanid-D)	Inotrope
Dexamethasone (Decadron)	Dexamethasone (Decadron, Hexadrol)	Steroid
Dextrose 50%	Dextrose 50%	Raises blood sugar
Diazepam (Valium, Diazemuls)	Diazepam (Valium)	Sedative, anticonvulsant
Digoxin (Lanoxin)	Digoxin (Lanoxin)	Inotrope
Dihydrocodeine (DF 118)	Dihydrocodeine (Paracodin)	Analgesic
Dobutamine (Dobutrex)	Dobutamine (Dobutrex)	Inotrope
Dopamine (Intropin)	Dopamine (Intropin)	Inotrope

British name	American name	Effects
Doxapram (Dopram)	Doxapram (Dopram)	Respiratory stimulant
Droperidol (Droleptan)	Droperidol (Inapsine)	Sedative, anti-emetic, α-blocker
Dysopyramide (Rhythmodan, Norpace)	Dysopyramide (Norpace)	Anti-dysrhythmic
Edrophonium (Tensilon)	Edrophonium (Tensilon)	Anticholinesterase
Ephedrine	Ephedrine	Vasopressor
Ergometrine	Ergometrine (Ergonovine)	Uterine constrictor
Flecainide (Tambocor)	Not available	Anti-arrhythmic
Flumazenil (Anexate)	Not available	Benzodiazepine antagonist
Frusemide (Lasix)	Furosemide (Lasix)	Diuretic
Gallamine (Flaxedil)	Gallamine (Flaxedil)	Muscle relaxant
Gentamicin (Genticin, Cidomycin)	Gentamicin (Garamycin)	Antibiotic
Glycopyrronium bromide (Robinul)	Glycopyrrolate (Robinul)	Anticholinergic
Heparin (Pularin)	Heparin	Anticoagulant
Hydralazine (Apresoline)	Hydralazine (Apresoline)	Hypotensive agent
Hydrocortisone	Hydrocortisone (Solu-cortef)	Steroid
Hyoscine (scopolamine)	Scopolamine (hyoscine)	Anticholinergic
Insulin	Insulin	Reduces blood sugar
Isoprenaline	Isoproterenol (Isuprel)	Inotrope
Ketamine (Ketalar)	Ketamine (Ketalar)	Induction agent
Labetalol (Trandate)	Labetalol	α- and β-blocker
Lignocaine (Xylocaine)	Lidocaine (Xylocaine)	Local anaesthetic, anti-dysrhythmic
Lorazepam (Ativan)	Lorazepam (Ativan)	Sedative
Meptazinol (Meptid)	Not available	Analgesic
Metaraminol (Aramine)	Metaraminol (Aramine)	Vasopressor
Methoxamine (Vasoxine)	Methoxamine (Vasoxyl)	Vasopressor
Methyl prednisolone (Solumedrone)	Methyl prednisolone (Solumedrone)	Steroid
Metoclopramide (Maxalon, Primperan)	Metoclopramide (Reglan)	Anti-emetic
Metronidazole (Flagyl, Zadstat)	Metronidazole (Flagyl)	Antibiotic
Midazolam (Hypnovel)	Midazolam (Versed)	Sedative
Morphine	Morphine	Analgesic
Nalbuphine (Nubain)	Nalbuphine (Nubain)	Analgesic
Naloxone (Narcan)	Naloxone (Narcan)	Opiate antagonist
Neostigmine (Prostigmin)	Neostigmine (Prostigmin)	Anticholinesterase
Nitroglycerin (Tridil)	Nitroglycerin	Hypotensive agent
Nitroprusside (Nipride)	Nitroprusside (Nipride)	Hypotensive agent
Oxytocin (Syntocinon)	Oxytocin (Pitocin, Syntocinon)	Uterine contraction

British name	American name	Effects
Pancuronium (Pavulon)	Pancuronium (Pavulon)	Muscle relaxant
Papaveretum (Omnopon)	No approved name (Pantopon)	Analgesic
Paracetamol (Panadol)	Acetaminophen (Phenaphen, Tempra)	Analgesic
Pentazocine (Fortral)	Pentazocine (Talwin)	Analgesic
Perphenazine (Fentazin)	Perphenazine (Trilafon)	Anti-emetic, antihistamine
Pethidine	Meperidine (Demerol)	Analgesic
Phenindione (Dindevan)	Phenindione (Hedulin)	Anticoagulant
Phenobarbitone (Luminal)	Phenobarbital (Luminal)	Anticonvulsant, sedative
Phentolamine (Rogitine)	Phentolamine (Rogitine)	α-blockade
Physostigmine (Eserine)	Physostigmine (Antilirium)	Anticholinesterase
Potassium chloride	Potassium chloride	Potassium replacement
Potassium iodide	Potassium iodide	Iodine replacement
Prilocaine (Citanest)	Prilocaine (Citanest)	Local anaesthetic
Procyclidine (Kemadrin)	Procyclidine (Kemadrin)	Anti-Parkinsonism
Propofol (Diprivan)	Not available	Induction agent
Propranolol (Inderal)	Propranolol (Inderal)	β-blockade
Promazine (Sparine)	Promazine (Sparine)	Anti-emetic
Protamine sulphate	Protamine sulfate	Reversal of heparin
Salbutamol (Ventolin)	Albuterol (Proventil, Ventolin)	Bronchodilator
Sodium valproate (Epilim)	Valproic acid (Depakene)	Anticonvulsant
Suxamethonium (Scoline, Anectine)	Succinylcholine chloride (Anectine, Quelicin)	Muscle relaxant
Tranexamic acid (Cyklokapron)	Not available	Antifibrinolysis
Trimetaphan (Arfonad)	Trimetaphan (Arfonad)	Hypotensive agent
Tubocurarine (Tubarine)	Tubocurarine (Curare)	Muscle relaxant
Vecuronium (Norcuron)	Vecuronium (Norcuron)	Muscle relaxant
Verapamil (Cordilox)	Verapamil (Isoptin, Calan)	Antidysrhythmic agent
Vitamin K (Konakion, Synka-Vit)	Phytonadione (Konakion, Aquamephyton)	Vitamin K replacement

Intravenous fluids

Compound sodium lactate (Hartmann's solution)	Lactated Ringer's solution
Dextran 40 (Rheomacrodex)	Dextran 40 (Gentran 40, LMD 10%, Rheomacrodex)
Dextran 70 (Macrodex)	Dextran 70 (Macrodex)
Dextrose 4%/sodium chloride 0.18%	Dextrose 4%/sodium chloride 0.18%
Dextrose 5%	Dextrose 5%
Hetastarch 6% (Hespan)	Hetastarch 6% (Hespan)
Human plasma protein fraction	Human plasma protein fraction (Plasmanate, Plasma-plex, plasmatein, Protenate)
Polygeline colloid 3.5% (Haemaccel)	Not available
Sodium bicarbonate 4.2%, 8.4%	Sodium bicarbonate 4.2%, 8.4%
Sodium chloride 0.18, 0.9, 1.8%	Sodium chloride 0.18%, 0.9%, 1.8%
Sodium chloride 0.18% or 0.45% in Dextrose 5%	

Bladder irrigation fluids

Glycine (aminoacetic acid)	Glycine (aminoacetic acid)
Sodium chloride 0.9%	Sodium chloride 0.9%

Cylinders
In addition to the above drugs, cylinders of oxygen, nitrous oxide, a 50:50 mixture of nitrous oxide and oxygen (Entonox) and a helium-oxygen mixture (helium 80%, oxygen 20%) should be available.

Appendix B. Translations of Standard Recovery Phrases

English	Open your mouth	Breathe deeply	Have you pain?	Your operation went well	Time to wake up
Arabic	Iftah fammak	Nafass shadeed	Fee alum?	Ama lia nagahet	Iss ha
Dutch	Open uw mond	Diep ademhalen	Heeft u pijn?	Alles is goed	Wakker worden
French	Ouvrez la bouche	Respirez profondément	Est-ce que vous avez mal?	Votre opération s'est bien passée	Reveillez-vous
German	Mund öffnen	Tief atmen	Tut es weh?	Die Operation ist gelungen	Aufwachen
Greek	Aneekse to stoma su	Anapnevse vathia	Echees pono?	El enhirissi sou pigay kala	Ohra na ksipnisis
Hindi/Urdu	Apna moonh kholiay	Lamba sans lee-jaye	Apko kaheen darad hay	Apka aperation theek ho gayahay?	Abb jaag jao
Italian	Aprite la bocca	Respirare profondamente	Avete dolore?	La vostra operazione e andata bene	E ora di svegliarvi
Japanese	Kuchi-o aitè	Shinkokyu-o shittay	Itami-ga arimasu-ka	Shujutsu-wa seiko desu	May-o aitè
Portuguese	Abra la boca	Respire fundo	Esta com dor?	A operacao foi bem	Acorde!
Spanish	Abra la boca	Respire profondamente	Tienes dolor?	Tu operacion a salido buen	Despiertese
Swedish	Oeppna munnen	Andas djupt	Har du Värk?	Din operation gick bra	Tid att vakna

Subject Index